CHILD AND ADOLESCENT PSYCHIATRY FOR PEDIATRICIANS

DR. MURAD BAKHT

MBBS (DAC), DCH (IRL), DTM&H (UK),
Dip Child Psych (C), FRCP (C)

Consultant Child and Adolescent Psychiatrist,

Brampton Civic Hospital, Brampton, Ontario,

Assistant Clinical Professor, McMaster
University, Hamilton, Ontario,

Canada

Editor: Farah Islam, PhD

Child and Adolescent Psychiatry for Pediatricians
Copyright © 2020 by Murad Bakht, FRCP (C)

All rights reserved. No part of this publication may be reproduced, distributed, or transmitted in any form or by any means, including photocopying, recording, or other electronic or mechanical methods, without the prior written permission of the author, except in the case of brief quotations embodied in critical reviews and certain other non-commercial uses permitted by copyright law.

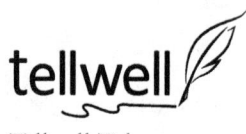

Tellwell Talent
www.tellwell.ca

ISBN
978-0-2288-2692-7 (Hardcover)
978-0-2288-2691-0 (Paperback)
978-0-2288-2693-4 (eBook)

This book is dedicated in memory of my parents

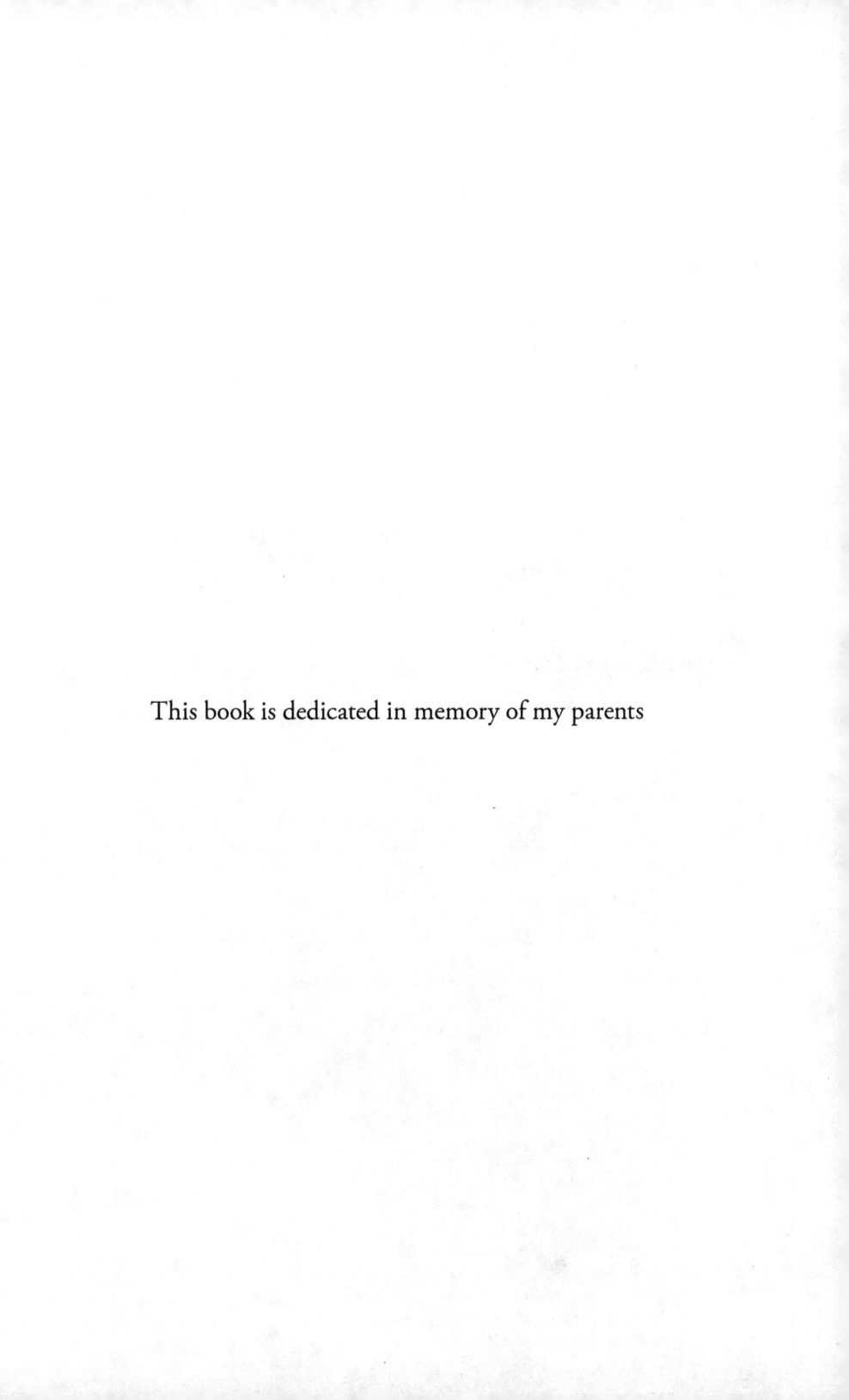

Acknowledgements

I acknowledge editor Dr. Farah Islam, hospital librarian Janice Thompson, and my family for their support.

Preface

Psychosocial problems are common health concerns in children and adolescents. Therefore, it is essential for pediatricians to be able to identify psychiatric disorders in childhood.

The lack of training in child psychiatry is still evident in many pediatric residency programs worldwide, including in developed countries such as the United States.[1] As recently as 2013, 65% of pediatricians surveyed by the American Academy of Pediatrics indicated they lacked training in recognizing and treating mental health problems.[2] This shortcoming adversely affects their knowledge, attitudes, and practices in childhood psychiatric disorders.[3] The inclusion of training in child psychiatry as a major part of all pediatrics academic curriculums and residency training programs would bridge the gap of this shortcoming. It is expected that the objectives of training in pediatrics residency programs include knowledge in children/adolescent mental health.[4]

---

[1] Behavioral and emotional problems among young preschool children in pediatric care; prevalence and pediatricians' recognition. Pediatric practice research group: J. V. Lavigne et al., Pediatrics 1993; March 91(3):649-655
[2] Pediatric Residency education and the behavioral and mental health crisis: A call for action; Julia A. McMillan et al., Pediatrics vol 139 no-1 January 2017
[3] Assessment of pediatricians need for training in child psychiatry; Fahad D AL – Osaimi et al J Fam Community medicine 2008;15(2):71-75
[4] Objective of training in Pediatrics Royal College of Physicians and Surgeons of Canada, 2008

Teaching child and adolescent psychiatry to pediatric residents for several years, I became interested in writing a book for pediatricians. This short book will cover topics in child psychiatry that are commonly faced by pediatricians in their day-to-day practice. In addition to pediatricians, it is my hope that pediatric residents, pediatric nurses, social workers, and psychologists will also find this book a useful resource.

Table of Contents

1. BASIC CONCEPTS IN MENTAL HEALTH

    OBJECTIVES 1
    DEFINITION OF MENTAL HEALTH............................1
    WHAT IS A MENTAL DISORDER? 1
    WHAT CAUSES MENTAL DISORDERS?......................1
    WHAT POPULATIONS ARE COMMONLY
    AFFECTED BY MENTAL DISORDERS?........................2
    HOW DO MENTAL DISORDERS AFFECT PEOPLE? ..2
    CONCLUSION...3

2. INFANT PSYCHIATRY

    OBJECTIVES 5
    IDEAL PRENATAL ENVIRONMENT 5
    MATERNAL AGE 5
    MATERNAL HEALTH AND NUTRITION 6
    DURATION OF MALNUTRITION 6
    PRENATAL HEALTH CARE..6
    CRITICAL PERIOD IN PRENATAL DEVELOPMENT.7
    TERATOGENS AND THEIR EFFECT...........................7
    MATERNAL DISEASES 8
    PRESCRIPTION AND OVER-THE-COUNTER
    (OTC) DRUGS..8
    MATERNAL STRESS 8
    FETAL ALCOHOL EFFECTS 9
    FETAL ALCOHOL SYNDROME (FAS) 9

HUMAN IMMUNODEFICIENCY VIRUS (HIV) 10
DIAGNOSTIC CLASSIFICATION OF
MENTAL HEALTH AND DEVELOPMENTAL
DISORDERS OF INFANCY AND EARLY
CHILDHOOD (DC: 0–3) 11
    Axis I: Primary Diagnoses of the Child 11
    Axis II: Parent-Child Relationship Problems 11
    Axis III: Physical, Neurological Disorders 11
    Axis IV: Psychosocial Stressors 12
    Axis V: Functional-Emotional Development Level 12
ASSESSMENT OF INFANTS AND YOUNG
CHILDREN 12
Management: 14
CONCLUSION 15

3. ESSENTIALS OF PSYCHIATRIC EVALUATION OF CHILDREN AND ADOLESCENTS

OBJECTIVES 18
ESSENTIAL CONCEPTS 18
SPECIAL CONSIDERATIONS IN EVALUATING
CHILDREN 19
COMPONENTS OF A THOROUGH
PSYCHIATRIC EVALUATION 20
INTERVIEW TECHNIQUES 20
PSYCHIATRIC INTERVIEW 21
FAMILY HISTORY 22
PREGNANCY, BIRTH AND
DEVELOPMENTAL MILESTONES 22
MENTAL-STATUS EXAMINATION 23
THOUGHT PROCESS 23
THOUGHT CONTENT 24
PERCEPTUAL DISTURBANCE 25
SENSORIUM (level of consciousness) 25

COGNITIVE FUNCTION 25
MINI MENTAL-STATE EXAM 26
JUDGMENT AND INSIGHT 26
FORMULATION 26
DIAGNOSIS 27
INVESTIGATION PROPOSED 27
MANAGEMENT 28
CONCLUSION 28

4. INTELLECTUAL DISABILITY

OBJECTIVES 30
DEFINITION 30
EPIDEMIOLOGY 30
CAUSES OF INTELLECTUAL DISABILITY 31
SYMPTOMS OF INTELLECTUAL DISABILITY 31
LEVELS OF INTELLECTUAL DISABILITY 32
ASSESSMENT 34
TREATMENT OPTIONS FOR INTELLECTUAL
DISABILITY 34
LONG-TERM OUTCOME 35
CONCLUSION 35
ONLINE RESOURCES 36

5. THE AUTISM SPECTRUM DISORDERS

OBJECTIVE 37
INTRODUCTION 37
DSM-5 DIAGNOSTIC CRITERIA OF AUTISM
SPECTRUM DISORDER 37
DSM-5 DIAGNOSTIC CRITERIA OF SOCIAL
(PRAGMATIC) COMMUNICATION DISORDER 38
EPIDEMIOLOGY OF ASD 39
ETIOLOGY OF ASDs 39
DEVELOPMENTAL WARNING SIGNS OF ASD 40

CLINICAL COURSE OF ASD 41
DIFFERENTIAL DIAGNOSIS OF AUTISM
SPECTRUM DISORDER... 41
COMORBID MENTAL DISORDERS 42
EVALUATION FOR CHILDREN WITH ASD
(CLINICAL HISTORY) 42
MANAGEMENT OF ASD 43
CONCLUSION 46

6. ATTENTION DEFICIT HYPERACTIVITY DISORDER

OBJECTIVES 48
INTRODUCTION 48
EPIDEMIOLOGY OF ADHD 49
CAUSE OF ADHD 49
DSM-5 DIAGNOSTIC CRITERIA FOR ADHD 49
ADHD SYMPTOMS MANIFEST
THROUGHOUT LIFE 51
CHILDHOOD ADHD COMMON CO-
MORBIDITIES 51
ADHD DIAGNOSTIC ASSESSMENT TECHNIQUES 51
ADHD DIFFERENTIAL DIAGNOSIS 51
RISKS OF NOT TREATING CHILD AND
ADOLESCENT ADHD 52
ADHD TREATMENT CHOICES 53
ADHD PHARMACOTHERAPY TREATMENT
OPTIONS 53
ADVANTAGES OF LONG-ACTING
STIMULANT FORMULATIONS 54
AREAS OF CONCERN AND CONTROVERSY
WITH STIMULANT USE AND ADVERSE EFFECTS 55
SIDE-EFFECT MANAGEMENT STRATEGIES 55
RECOMMENDATION FOR STARTING AND
MAXIMUM DOSES OF STIMULANTS 56

PSYCHOSOCIAL TREATMENT OF ADHD 58
TREATMENT OF ADHD AND COMORBIDITY 60
COURSE AND PROGNOSIS OF ADHD 61
CONCLUSION 62

7. OPPOSITIONAL DEFIANT DISORDER

OBJECTIVES 66
INTRODUCTION 66
CHARACTERISTICS OF THE INFLEXIBLE-
EXPLOSIVE CHILD 66
SOME OBSERVATIONS 67
ADDITIONAL OBSERVATIONS 67
EPIDEMIOLOGY 68
ETIOLOGY 68
DIAGNOSTIC CRITERIA OF ODD (DSM-5) 68
SOME PROBLEMS WITH ODD DIAGNOSIS 69
DIFFERENTIAL DIAGNOSIS 69
COMORBIDITY 69
DYNAMICS OF ODD 70
AACAP GUIDELINES FOR ASSESSMENT AND
TREATMENT OF ODD 71
PSYCHOSOCIAL MANAGEMENT 72
PHARMACOLOGICAL INTERVENTION 73
NATURAL COURSE OF ODD 73
PREVENTION OF ODD 73
CONCLUSION 74

8. CONDUCT DISORDER

OBJECTIVES 76
INTRODUCTION 76
DSM-5 DIAGNOSTIC CRITERIA FOR CD 76
EPIDEMIOLOGY 77
ETIOLOGY 78

RISK FACTORS 78
PROTECTIVE FACTORS 79
ESSENTIALS OF ASSESSMENT OF CD 80
DIFFERENTIAL DIAGNOSIS 80
COMORBIDITY OF CONDUCT DISORDER 81
CRITICAL ISSUES IN TREATMENT PLANNING 81
MANAGEMENT 82
PROMISING TREATMENT STRATEGIES 83
MEDICATION MANAGEMENT OF CD 83
COURSE OF CD 83
PROGNOSIS 84
CONCLUSION 85

9. TIC DISORDERS

OBJECTIVES 87
CHARACTERISTIC FEATURES 87
TOURETTE'S SYNDROME 87
TREATMENT 88
EDUCATION 88

10. FETAL ALCOHOL SYNDROME

OBJECTIVES 90
INTRODUCTION 90
FAS WITH CONFIRMED MATERNAL
ALCOHOL EXPOSURE 91
PARTIAL OR ATYPICAL FAS WITH
CONFIRMED MATERNAL ALCOHOL EXPOSURE . 91
SCREENING FOR ALCOHOL USE/ABUSE 92
PREVENTION OF FAS 93
COMORBIDITY 94
TREATMENT FOR FAS CHILDREN 95
CONCLUSION 95

11. COMMON ANXIETY DISORDERS IN CHILDHOOD AND ADOLESCENCE

OBJECTIVES 97
INTRODUCTION 97
SEPARATION ANXIETY DISORDER (SAD) 98
    Essential Concepts of SAD 98
    Epidemiology 98
    Etiology 98
    Assessment 99
    Diagnosis 99
    Management of SAD 99
SELECTIVE MUTISM 100
    Epidemiology 100
    Treatment 101
SSRI 101
PANIC DISORDER 101
    Epidemiology 101
    Diagnosis 101
    Treatment 102
    Prognosis 102
AGORAPHOBIA 102
GENERALIZED ANXIETY DISORDER (GAD) 103
    Epidemiology 103
    Diagnosis 103
    Treatment 103
    Prognosis 104
SPECIFIC PHOBIA 104
    Epidemiology 104
    Features 104
    Diagnosis 104
    Types 104
    Treatment 105
SOCIAL ANXIETY DISORDER 105

Epidemiology 105
Symptoms 105
Treatment 105
Prognosis 106
POST-TRAUMATIC STRESS DISORDER (PTSD) 106
Epidemiology 106
Diagnosis 106
Treatment 107
CONCLUSION 107

12. CHILDHOOD AND ADOLESCENT DEPRESSION

OBJECTIVES 109
INTRODUCTION 109
EPIDEMIOLOGY OF DEPRESSION 110
ETIOLOGY OF DEPRESSION 110
CLINICAL PRESENTATION 111
DSM-5 DIAGNOSTIC CRITERIA FOR
DEPRESSION 111
SUBTYPES OF DEPRESSION 111
PERSISTENT DEPRESSIVE DISORDER
"DYSTHYMIA" 112
RISK FACTORS FOR DEPRESSION 112
ASSESSMENT OF DEPRESSION 113
DIFFERENTIAL DIAGNOSIS OF DEPRESSION 114
MEDICAL DISORDERS 115
COMORBIDITY OF DEPRESSION 115
CONTROVERSY ABOUT THE USE OF
ANTIDEPRESSANTS IN CHILDREN AND
ADOLESCENTS 116
CLINICAL RECOMMENDATIONS FOR USE
OF ANTIDEPRESSANTS 116
MEDICATION TREATMENT FOR DEPRESSION ... 117
SIDE EFFECTS OF ANTIDEPRESSANTS 117

PRINCIPLES OF TREATMENT FOR DEPRESSION 118
DEPRESSION AND SUICIDALITY 119
COURSE OF DEPRESSION 120
PROGNOSIS OF DEPRESSION 121
PREVENTION OF DEPRESSION 121
CONCLUSION 122

13. PEDIATRIC BIPOLAR MOOD DISORDER

OBJECTIVES 124
INTRODUCTION 124
DSM-5 DIAGNOSTIC CRITERIA OF
DISRUPTIVE MOOD DISREGULATION
DISORDER 125
TREATMENT APPROACH FOR DISRUPTIVE
MOOD DYSREGULATION DISORDER 126
MANIA: DSM-5 CRITERIA 126
HYPOMANIA DSM-5 CRITERIA 127
MAJOR DEPRESSIVE EPISODE DSM-5 CRITERIA .. 127
CYCLOTHYMIC DISORDER 128
EPIDEMIOLOGY 129
WHY IS BIPOLAR DISORDER DIFFICULT TO
DIAGNOSE IN CHILDREN AND YOUTH? 129
RISK FACTORS THAT MAY PREDICT
EVENTUAL MANIC EPISODE 129
PARENT-REPORTED SYMPTOMS IN
CHILDREN WHO MAY ULTIMATELY
BECOME BIPOLAR 130
FEATURES UNIQUE TO YOUTH IN BIPOLAR
ILLNESS 130
ASSESSMENT 130
DIFFERENTIAL DIAGNOSIS OF BIPOLAR
DISORDER 131

AVAILABLE TREATMENT OF BIPOLAR
DISORDER... 131
TREATMENT OF MANIA 132
MANAGEMENT OF MIXED, MANIC AND
RAPID CYCLIC MOOD DISORDER 132
BIPOLAR DISORDER—DEPRESSION 132
TREATMENT RESISTANCE ISSUES 132
ENHANCING COMPLIANCE..................................... 133
TREATMENT STRATEGY: MOVING BEYOND
EPISODES... 133
PSYCHOSOCIAL MANAGEMENT 133
PEDIATRIC BIPOLAR: OUTCOMES 133
CONCLUSION... 134

14. FIRST-EPISODE PSYCHOSIS

OBJECTIVES 136
INTRODUCTION... 136
DEFINITION OF FIRST-EPISODE PSYCHOSIS 136
FACTS ABOUT PSYCHOSIS....................................... 137
GOALS OF EARLY DETECTION AND
INTERVENTION 137
PRODROMAL FEATURES.. 137
EARLY WARNING SIGN OF FIRST-EPISODE
PSYCHOSIS 138
SYMPTOMS OF PSYCHOSIS 138
DIFFERENTIAL DIAGNOSIS OF FIRST-
EPISODE PSYCHOSIS 138
ASSESSMENT OF FIRST-EPISODE PSYCHOSIS 139
COMPREHENSIVE TREATMENT OF FIRST-
EPISODE PSYCHOSIS 140
SIMPLIFICATION OF TREATMENT REGIMES 140
FIRST-EPISODE DOSING OF ANTIPSYCHOTICS... 140
PSYCHOSOCIAL MANAGEMENT 141

ISSUES OF TREATMENT ADHERENCE IN
FIRST-EPISODE PSYCHOSIS 141
IDENTIFICATION OF NON-ADHERENCE IN
TREATMENT 141
MEDICATION-RELATED FACTORS FOR
NONCOMPLIANCE 142
FUNCTIONAL RECOVERY FROM FIRST-
EPISODE PSYCHOSIS 142
WHAT PREDICTS CLINICAL AND
FUNCTIONAL OUTCOME? 143
PREVENTING PROGRESSION OF DISEASE
AND IMPROVING OUTCOME 143
CONCLUSION 144

15. EATING DISORDERS

OBJECTIVES 146
INTRODUCTION 146
ANOREXIA NERVOSA 146
EPIDEMIOLOGY OF ANOREXIA NERVOSA 147
DSM-5 CRITERIA FOR ANOREXIA NERVOSA 147
ANOREXIA NERVOSA SUBTYPES 147
ASSOCIATED FEATURES 147
RISK FACTORS 148
BULIMIA NERVOSA (BN) 148
DSM-5 CRITERIA FOR BN 149
ASSOCIATED FEATURES 149
BINGE EATING DISORDER 150
OBESITY 150
COMORBIDITY IN EATING DISORDERS 150
MEDICAL ASSESSMENT 151
LABORATORY TESTS 151
MULTIMODAL TREATMENT OF EATING
DISORDERS 152

MEDICATIONS 153
RELAPSE PREVENTION 153
PROGNOSIS FOR AN AND BN 154
CONCLUSION 154

16. PICA

OBJECTIVES 156
DIAGNOSTIC CRITERIA 156
PREVALENCE 156
COURSE 156
RISK AND PROGNOSTIC FACTORS 157
CULTURE-RELATED DIAGNOSTIC ISSUES 157
DIAGNOSTIC MARKERS 157
DIFFERENTIAL DIAGNOSIS 157
COMORBIDITY 157
TREATMENT 158
CONCLUSION 158

17. RUMINATION DISORDER

OBJECTIVES 160
DEFINITION 160
EPIDEMIOLOGY 160
ETIOLOGY 160
DEVELOPMENT AND COURSE 160
RISK FACTORS 161
ASSOCIATED FEATURES 161
DIFFERENTIAL DIAGNOSIS 161
TREATMENT 161
OUTCOME 161
CONCLUSION 161

18. ENCOPRESIS

OBJECTIVES 163
DEFINITION 163
TYPES 163
EPIDEMIOLOGY 163
ETIOLOGY 164
ASSESSMENT 164
MANAGEMENT 165
OUTCOME 165
CONCLUSION 165

19. ENURESIS

OBJECTIVES 167
DEFINITION 167
TYPES OF ENURESIS 167
EPIDEMIOLOGY 168
ETIOLOGY 168
ASSESSMENT 168
MANAGEMENT 169
CONCLUSION 170

20. OBSESSIVE-COMPULSIVE AND RELATED DISORDERS

OBJECTIVES 172
OBSESSIVE-COMPULSIVE DISORDER 172
    Definition 172
    Epidemiology 172
    Diagnosis 172
    Treatment 173
    Prognosis 173
    Conclusion 174
TRICHOTILLOMANIA 174
    Diagnostic Criteria 174

Clinical Presentation 174
Prevalence 174
Risk Factors 175
Culture-Related Issues 175
Diagnosis 175
Differential Diagnosis 175
Comorbidities 176
Functional Consequences 176
Treatment 176
Prognosis 176
Conclusion 177
BODY DYSMORPHIC DISORDER 177
Definition 177
HOARDING DISORDER 177
Definition 177
EXCORIATION (SKIN-PICKING) DISORDER 178
Definition 178

21. PRINCIPLES OF PSYCHIATRIC TREATMENT

OBJECTIVES 180
INTRODUCTION 180
PSYCHOPHARMACOLOGY 180
ESSENTIALS FOR THE USE OF
PHARMACOTHERAPY 181
MAJOR CLASSES OF MEDICATIONS USED IN
PSYCHIATRY 181
Stimulants 181
Antidepressants 182
Therapeutic use of Antidepressants 182
Tricyclic Antidepressants (TCA) 183
Serotonin Reuptake Inhibitors (SSRI) 183
Atypical Antidepressants 183
Mood Stabilizers 184

Anxiolytics 184
Antipsychotics 185
ELECTROCONVULSIVE THERAPY (ECT) 185
PSYCHOTHERAPY 186
COMMON TYPES OF PSYCHOTHERAPY 186
SPECIFIC THERAPIES FOR SPECIFIC DISORDERS 186
PARENT MANAGEMENT TRAINING 188
CONCLUSION 188

22. CHILD ABUSE AND NEGLECT

OBJECTIVES 190
INTRODUCTION 190
DEFINITION OF CHILD MALTREATMENT 191
Physical abuse 191
Sexual abuse 191
Child neglect 191
Emotional abuse (psychological/verbal/mental abuse) .. 191
GLOBAL PREVALENCE OF CHILD
MALTREATMENT AND ABUSE 191
CANADIAN INCIDENCE REPORT OF CHILD
ABUSE 192
PHYSICAL ABUSE 192
INDICATOR FOR RISK OF SEXUAL ABUSE 193
EMOTIONAL ABUSE 193
MUNCHAUSEN'S SYNDROME BY PROXY 194
RISK FACTORS FOR CHILD MALTREATMENT 195
INDICATORS FOR RISK OF PHYSICAL ABUSE 196
PARENTAL CHARACTERISTICS FOR
PHYSICAL ABUSE 196
ABUSE CIRCUMSTANCES 196
COMMON SITES FOR ACCIDENTAL INJURY 197
SITES OF POSSIBLE NON-ACCIDENTAL INJURY .. 198
PSYCHOSOCIAL IMPACT IN ABUSED CHILDREN 198

INDICATORS OF NEGLECT.................................. 198
PARENTAL CHARACTERISTICS FOR NEGLECT .. 199
PARENTAL CIRCUMSTANCES OF CHRONIC
NEGLECT 199
CHILD CHARACTERISTICS FOR NEGLECT.......... 200
EFFECT OF NEGLECT IN CHILDHOOD................. 200
EXTREME EFFECT OF NEGLECT IN
CHILDHOOD.. 200
ADULT CONSEQUENCE OF CHILDHOOD
NEGLECT 201
DOMESTIC VIOLENCE... 201
EFFECTS ON CHILD WITNESSES OF
DOMESTIC VIOLENCE.. 201
ASSESSMENT OF SUSPECTED ABUSE OR
NEGLECT 202
PHYSICAL EXAMINATION OF SUSPECTED
ABUSE OR NEGLECT 203
MANAGEMENT OF CHILD ABUSE AND
NEGLECT 203
PROTECTIVE FACTORS TO PREVENT
CHILD MALTREATMENT.................................... 204
CONCLUSION... 205

23. FAILURE TO THRIVE (FTT)

OBJECTIVES 207
NEGATIVE IMPACT OF FAILURE TO THRIVE
IN CHILDREN 207
IDENTIFICATION OF FAILURE TO THRIVE 207
POVERTY CORRELATES WITH FTT 208
EARLY INTERVENTION...................................... 208
HOME INTERVENTION...................................... 208
PREVENTION OF FAILURE TO THRIVE 208
CONCLUSION... 209

24. PEDIATRIC SOMATIZATION

OBJECTIVES 211
EPIDEMIOLOGY OF SOMATIZATION 211
SOMATIZATION WITH CO-OCCURRING
ANXIETY 211
NEGATIVE IMPACT OF SOMATIZATION 212
TREATMENT SOMATIZATION 212
FAMILY INTERVENTION OF SOMATIZATION 213
CONCLUSION 213

25. LEARNING DISORDERS

OBJECTIVES 215
INTRODUCTION 215
INTELLECTUAL DEVELOPMENTAL DISORDER .. 215
GLOBAL DEVELOPMENTAL DELAY 216
DUAL DIAGNOSIS 216
ASSESSMENT 216
TYPES OF DISABILITIES 217
SERVICE MODEL 217
SPECIALIZED SERVICE REQUIREMENTS
AND CARE PLAN 217
RESIDENTIAL SERVICE 218
COMMUNITY PARTICIPATION 219
CONCLUSION 219

26. JUVENILE SUBSTANCE ABUSE

OBJECTIVES 221
INTRODUCTION 221
EPIDEMIOLOGY 221
FINDINGS FROM THE STUDENT DRUG USE
SURVEY 2009, ONTARIO, CANADA 222
RISK FACTORS FOR DEVELOPING
SUBSTANCE-ABUSE PROBLEMS 223

PROTECTIVE FACTORS 224
STAGES OF SUBSTANCE USE 224
  Terminology 225
PATHWAYS OF JUVENILE SUBSTANCE ABUSE 225
DYNAMIC ISSUES 226
JUVENILE SUBSTANCE ABUSE AND
PSYCHIATRIC COMORBIDITIES 226
CONSIDER SCREENING FOR SUBSTANCE
ABUSE..227
C-R-A-F-F-T Substance Abuse Screening Questionnaires.227
ASSESSMENT FOR SUBSTANCE ABUSE 228
MULTIMODAL TREATMENT OF
SUBSTANCE USE DISORDERS......................................228
PSYCHOPHARMACOLOGICAL STRATEGIES 229
PREVENTION...229
CONCLUSION..230

27. INTERNET, VIDEO GAMING, AND GAMBLING ADDICTION IN ADOLESCENTS

OBJECTIVES 233
INTRODUCTION...233
INTERNET ADDICTION 234
  Why does excessive internet use occur? 234
  Diagnostic criteria for identifying internet addiction....234
  Risk factor for problematic internet use.........................235
  Negative impact of internet addiction 235
  Internet addiction, and comorbidity...............................235
  Treatment for internet addiction 235
VIDEO-GAME ADDICTION 236
  Reasons why males play
  video games more than females.......................................236
  Diagnostic criteria for video-game addiction.................236
  Medical complication of video-game addiction............237

Social impact of video-game addiction..........................237
Treatment for video-game addiction 237
GAMBLING ADDICTION 238
Introduction 238
Epidemiology of gambling....................................238
Etiological factors of gambling.............................238
Risk factors for gambling addiction 238
Gambling and comorbidity....................................239
Pathological gambling and comorbidity.......................239
DSM-5 criteria for gambling disorders...........................239
Prevention of underage problem gambling.................240
Treatment for gambling addiction............................241
The McGill treatment paradigm...........................241
CONCLUSION...242

28. CYBERBULLYING

OBJECTIVES 244
SOCIAL MEDIA 244
SOCIAL MEDIA SITES..244
ROLE OF FRONTLINE CLINICIANS........................245
WHAT IS CYBERBULLYING? 245
HOW CYBERBULLIES OPERATE 245
A NEW FACE FOR AN OLD MONSTER...................246
TYPES OF CYBERBULLYING 246
EFFECTS 247
ADULT OUTCOMES OF CHILDHOOD
BULLYING 247
FACTORS CO-OCCURRING WITH
CYBERBULLYING AND SUICIDE............................247
IMPACT AT SCHOOL..248
CORRELATION BETWEEN CYBERBULLYING
AND SUICIDE 248
VICTIMS 249

REASONS CITED BY STUDENTS FOR NOT
REPORTING CYBERBULLYING TO SCHOOL 249
WARNING SIGNS 250
STATISTICS 250
INTERVENTIONS 251
ADDITIONAL INTERVENTIONS 251
ROLE OF FRONTLINE CLINICIANS 252
RISK ASSESSMENT OF BULLYING VICTIM 252
WHERE DO PARENTS FIT IN? 252
HOW SCHOOLS CAN HELP 253
ONLINE SAFETY 254
SOLUTIONS 254
ONLINE RESOURCES 255
CONCLUSION 255
INDEX 257

1. BASIC CONCEPTS IN MENTAL HEALTH

OBJECTIVES

This chapter will include a definition of mental health, common causes of mental disorders, populations affected by mental disorders, and how mental disorders impact an individual's daily functioning.

DEFINITION OF MENTAL HEALTH

Mental health can be defined as the psychological state of someone who is functioning at a satisfactory level of emotional and behavioural adjustment.

WHAT IS A MENTAL DISORDER?

A mental disorder is an illness with psychological or behavioural manifestations associated with impairment in functioning.

Each illness has characteristic signs and symptoms.

WHAT CAUSES MENTAL DISORDERS?

Genetic factors

Developmental disorders

Environmental factors

Stress

Life events
Family as a "pathogenic institution"
Medical illness

WHAT POPULATIONS ARE COMMONLY AFFECTED BY MENTAL DISORDERS?

Most major mental illness tends to manifest in the adolescent years.

Studies suggest that women are more susceptible to mental disorder than men, e.g., pre-menstrual period, puerperium, and following a hysterectomy. Also, women are less inhibited than men in discussing emotional problems, and while marriage seems to be a protective factor for men, it may place women at a greater risk for a mental disorder.

There is a strong relationship between social class and mental disorder: the lowest social classes are at a higher risk of mental disorders.

Suicide risk tends to increase with age.

Incidence of paranoia and depressive illness increases in middle age.

Transcultural studies reveal variations in concepts of health and disorder.

HOW DO MENTAL DISORDERS AFFECT PEOPLE?

Mental disorders may cause disturbance of thought, perception, mood, and behaviour.

Most common thought disturbance is delusion.

Most common perceptual disturbance is hallucination.

Mood (affect) is subject to a wide range of disturbances, from mania to depression and anxiety.

General behaviour and activity are also subject to a variety of disturbances.

CONCLUSION

The dimensions of mental health are diverse. Each illness has characteristic signs and symptoms. Gene and environment interactions are the most common causal factors of mental illness. Certain populations may be at a higher risk of mental illness than others.

REFERENCES

Jacobs, S. C., & Steiner, J. L. (Eds.). (2016). *Yale Textbook of Public Psychiatry*. New York, NY, USA: Oxford University Press.

Lyttle, J. (1986). *Mental Disorder: Its Care and Treatment*. London, UK: Bailliere Tindall.

Pilgrim, D., Rogers, A., & Pescosolido, B. A. (Eds.). (2011). *The SAGE Handbook of Mental Health and Illness*. London, UK: Sage Publications.

Thornicroft, G., & Szmukler, G. (Eds.). (2001). *Textbook of Community Psychiatry*. New York, NY, USA: Oxford University Press.

2. INFANT PSYCHIATRY

OBJECTIVES

This chapter will focus on infant psychiatry by looking at the prenatal environment, maternal age, health and nutrition, prenatal health care, critical period in prenatal development, teratogens and their effect, maternal diseases, prescription and over-the-counter drugs, maternal stress, alcohol use in pregnancy, fetal alcohol syndrome, HIV, and finally, assessment of infant and young children and their treatment.

IDEAL PRENATAL ENVIRONMENT

Well-developed amniotic sac

Cushion of amniotic fluid

Fully functioning placenta and umbilical cord

Adequate supply of oxygen and nutrients

Freedom from invading disease organisms and toxic agents

MATERNAL AGE

Greatest success rate is for mothers in their twenties

At greater risk: teenage mothers and mothers over 35–40 years old

For teenage mothers: their bodies may not yet be mature enough to conceive and sustain a healthy developing child

For older mothers: older ova (aged or damaged), also older bodies and differing hormonal balance could be factors

Older mothers have a greater risk of miscarriage and producing an infant with Down syndrome

Teenage and older mothers: miscarriages, stillbirths, congenital anomalies

MATERNAL HEALTH AND NUTRITION

Unbalanced diet, vitamin, protein, or other deficiencies

Deficiencies in the mother's digestive processes and overall metabolism

Low birth weight, smaller head size, smaller overall size of infant

Spontaneous abortion, premature birth, death of infant shortly after birth

Significant fetal malnutrition can predispose for adult disorders; hypertension, coronary heart disease, and thyroid disease, as well as schizophrenia

Reduced brain development in late fetal period or early infancy

DURATION OF MALNUTRITION

Mothers, by drawing on their own stored reserves, protect the fetus from the effects of short-term malnutrition.

Both mother and fetus thus appear to be capable of recovering from limited malnutrition.

If the period of fetal malnourishment has been relatively short, it can sometimes be compensated for by infant nutrition programs.

PRENATAL HEALTH CARE

Careful health history

Full medical examination

Counselling about potential risks and the avoidance of alcohol, tobacco, and illicit drugs

Advice about the value of regular physical exercise

Recommendations regarding good nutrition

Reduction of vaccine-preventable diseases (measles, diphtheria, meningitis) can lower infant mortality

CRITICAL PERIOD IN PRENATAL DEVELOPMENT

Many of the damaging effects on prenatal development can occur before the woman is even aware that she is pregnant.

Major abnormalities of the central nervous system or the heart may occur as a result of diseases the mother contracts or substances she ingests during the early embryonic period.

More frequently, the teratogen results in an increased risk of damage, which may occur in varying degrees or not at all.

Whether there is damage depends on a complex interaction of factors, including the amount and duration of exposure, the developmental stage of the fetus, the overall health of the mother, and genetic factors.

TERATOGENS AND THEIR EFFECT

A teratogen is a toxic agent of any kind that can potentially cause abnormalities in the developing child.

Drugs, diseases, hormones, blood factors, radiation, exposure to toxins in the workplace (e.g., lead, certain gases), along with maternal age, nutrition, stress, and type of prenatal care all play a part in the development of the embryo or fetus.

Some drugs and other chemicals can be turned into waste products and eliminated by the mother's mature body but not by the fetus.

There may still be other harmful environmental agents whose influences have not yet been determined.

MATERNAL DISEASES

Most kinds of bacteria do not cross a normal placental barrier.

Smaller organisms, such as many viruses, particularly rubella (German measles), herpes simplex, and many varieties of cold and flu viruses can cross the placental barrier.

Rubella can cause blindness, heart abnormalities, deafness, brain damage, or limb deformity.

Diseases may enter the child by one of three routes: directly through the placenta (rubella and HIV), indirectly through the amniotic fluid (syphilis and gonorrhea), and during labour and delivery (interchange of bodily fluids and perhaps blood).

PRESCRIPTION AND OVER-THE-COUNTER (OTC) DRUGS

A Michigan study of nearly 19,000 women found that they consumed an average of three prescription drugs during their pregnancies

Tetracycline (antibiotic): adverse effects on fetal teeth and bones

Anticonvulsants: structural malformations, growth delays, heart abnormalities, mild mental retardation, or speech irregularities

Oral contraceptives: malformation of the fetal sexual organs

Diethylstilbestrol (DES): daughters had a higher than normal incidence of vaginal cancer or cervical abnormalities; sons were sterile or prone to develop testicular cancer

MATERNAL STRESS

Infants of rhesus monkeys exposed to stress during pregnancy showed an abnormal physiological reaction to stress.

Also, infants of rhesus monkeys reared separately from their mother showed changes in levels of stress-related hormones.

There is a higher risk of substance use during pregnancy with maternal stress.

There is no evidence that mild, occasional stress causes problems.

FETAL ALCOHOL EFFECTS

Animal and human research make it clear that alcohol severely disrupts prenatal brain development in a variety of ways.

In the USA, 20% of newborns have had prenatal alcohol exposure.

One percent of newborns have obvious neurological problems, with a higher percentage of newborns having more subtle cognitive and behavioural problems.

FETAL ALCOHOL SYNDROME (FAS)

Unusual facial characteristics

Poor growth

Central nervous system problems (mental retardation, irritability, hyperactivity)

Third leading cause of mental retardation in the USA

The following FAS symptoms may not always be corrected after birth:

- Unusual facial characteristics
- Flattened nose
- Underdeveloped upper lip
- Poorly developed indentation above the upper lip
- Widely spaced eyes
- Flat cheekbones

- Growth retardation
- Low birth weight (LBW)
- Small head
- Smaller than average stature throughout life

Other symptoms:
- Significant impairment in attention
- Impairment in neuromotor functioning
- Disrupted attachment
- Disruption in social behaviour
- Neurological and behavioural problems:
  ○ Irritability
  ○ Reduced information processing speed
  ○ Lowered IQ
  ○ Motor difficulties
  ○ Problems with arithmetic and reading
- Heightened risk of nicotine, alcohol, and drug dependence

HUMAN IMMUNODEFICIENCY VIRUS (HIV)

Can cross the placenta

Infection by the mother's blood during delivery

Infection through breastfeeding

By 2002, an estimated 19.2 million women worldwide

Estimated 3.2 million children under age 15 (UNAIDS, 2002)

Highest concentration in Sub-Saharan Africa

Rate of transmission in Africa: 25%–35% (USA 15–25%)

Symptoms in infants:

- Failure to grow, even with treatment
- Repeated serious infections
- Brain development: problems in motor and cognitive development

DIAGNOSTIC CLASSIFICATION OF MENTAL HEALTH AND DEVELOPMENTAL DISORDERS OF INFANCY AND EARLY CHILDHOOD (DC: 0–3)

Axis I: Primary Diagnoses of the Child

Traumatic disorders

Affective disorders

Anxiety disorders

Mood disorders

Attachment disorders

Regulation disorders

Axis II: Parent-Child Relationship Problems

Over-involved parent relationship

Under-involved parent relationship

Anxious/tense relationship

Angry/hostile relationship with or without physical or sexual abuse

Axis III: Physical, Neurological Disorders

Physical diseases

Neurological problems

Diagnoses from physical therapists, language specialists, etc.

Axis IV: Psychosocial Stressors

Stress index: adoption, poverty, birth of sibling, violence (environment), abuse (emotional, physical, sexual), accidents, hospitalization, illness, loss of a loved one, etc.

Axis V: Functional-Emotional Development Level

ASSESSMENT OF INFANTS AND YOUNG CHILDREN

Assessing an infant or young child includes interviewing the parents and other adults in the child's environment (teacher, coach, family member).

Interviewing the parents:

- Child's current difficulties and reasons for referral
- Developmental history
- Cognitive and academic development
- Family relationships
- Peer relationships
- Physical development and medical history
- Emotional development and temperament (parents' response)
- Development of conscience and values
- Interests, hobbies, talents, and avocations
- Unusual circumstances
- Family and community background
- Parents as individuals and as a couple
- When adopted: circumstances, expectations, and feelings
- Parents' feelings about and involvement with the child
- Education and occupation

- Parents' history
- Community: neighbourhood, religion, culture

Psychiatric assessment of the infant/young child:
- Mental-status examination
- Child interviewing techniques: depend on the child's developmental, cognitive and linguistic level, the emotional difficulty of the issue being addressed, and the degree of rapport between child and clinician
- Physical appearance
- Manner of relating to examiner and parents
- Affect
- Coping mechanisms
- Orientation to time, place, person
- Motor behaviour, including activity level
- Quality of thinking and perception
- Speech and language
- Overall intelligence and fund of knowledge
- Attention, concentration, and impulsivity
- Neurological functioning
- Judgment and insight
- Preferred modes of communication
- Play techniques
- Imaginative play to communicate
- Clinician follows the sequences of play content, noting themes that emerge, points at which the child backs away from the storyline or shifts to a new sequence or activity,

and situations in which the child gets stuck or falls into a repetitive loop
- Observing the form of play, coordination and motor capacities, speech and language development, attention span, readiness to engage the interviewer, capacity of complex thought, and affective state
- Projective techniques:
  - Drawing pictures
  - Leaving the choice of subject up to the child or making a specific request
  - Asking which animal the child would most or least like to be
  - Three magic wishes
  - Asking the child to recount a dream, movie or book
- Direct questions:
  - Requires attention to the child's level of cognitive and linguistic development and regard for the effect of the question on the child's self-esteem
  - Phrase the question in language that is appropriate to the child's developmental level and verbal capacities
  - Open-ended questions

MANAGEMENT:
- Educating and supporting the parents
- Cognitive Behavioural Therapy (CBT)
- Family therapy
- Play-therapy, sensory stimulation, relaxation exercises, mindfulness
- Engage with the child (YouTube, music, exercises)

CONCLUSION

Multiple prenatal factors, including environment, toxins, maternal age, and health contributes to an infant or child's healthy development. The appropriate assessment of an infant or young child will identify any adversity and, accordingly, treatment can be provided.

REFERENCES

Brown, A. S., Susser, E. S., Butler, P. D., Andrews, R. R., Kaufmann, C. A., & Gorman, J. M. (1996). Neurobiological plausibility of prenatal nutritional deprivation as a risk factor for schizophrenia. *Journal of Nervous and Mental Disease, 184,* 71–85.

Centers for Disease Control and Prevention. Fourth Report on Human Exposure to Environmental Chemicals, Updated Tables, (January 2019). Atlanta, GA: U.S. Department of Health and Human Services, Centers for Disease Control and Prevention. https://www.cdc.gov/exposurereport/

Chiodo, L. M., Jacobson, S. W. & Jacobson, J. L. (2000). Neurodevelopmental effects of postnatal lead exposure at very low levels. *Neurotoxicology and Teratology, 26*(3), 359–371.

Craig, G. J. & Baucum, D. (Eds.). (2003). *Human Development* (9th ed.). Upper Saddle River, NJ, USA: Prentice-Hall.

Dalman, C., Allebeck, P., Cullberg, J., Grunewald, C., & Koester, M. (1999). Obstetric complications and the risk of schizophrenia: A longitudinal study of a national birth cohort. *Archives of General Psychiatry, 56,* 234–240.

DeHart, G., Sroufe, L. A., & Cooper, R. G. (Eds.). (2004). *Child Development: Its Nature and Course* (5th ed.). New York, NY, USA: McGraw-Hill Companies.

Diagnostic Classification of Mental Health and Developmental Disorders of Infancy and Early Childhood (DC: 0 –3R). (2005). ZERO TO THREE.

Guerri, C. (1998). Neuroanatomical and Neurophysiological Mechanisms Involved in Central Nervous System Dysfunctions Induced by Prenatal Alcohol Exposure. *Alcoholism: Clinical and Experimental Research, 22,* 304–312.

Kelly, S. J., Day, N., & Streissguth, A. P. (2000). Effects of prenatal alcohol exposure on social behavior in humans and other species. *Neurotoxicology and Teratology, 22*(2), 143–149.

Metcoff, J., Costiloe, J. P., Crosby, W., Bentle, L., et al. (1981). Maternal nutrition and fetal outcome. *American Journal of Clinical Nutrition, 34*(10), 708–721.

Msall, M. E., Bier, J. A., LaGasse, L., Tremont, M., & Lester, B. (1998). The vulnerable preschool child: the impact of biomedical and social risks on neurodevelopmental function. *Semin Pediatr Neurol., 5*(1):52–61.

Piper, J. M., Baum, C., & Kennedy, D. L. (1987). Prescription drug use before and during pregnancy in a Medicaid population. *Am J Obstet Gynecol., 157*(1), 148–156.

Sadock, B. J. (2006). *Kaplan and Sadock's Comprehensive Textbook of Psychiatry* (9th ed.). V. A. Sadock & P. Ruiz (Eds.). South Holland, Netherlands: Wolters Kluwer.

Sampson, P. D., Streissguth, A. P., Bookstein, F. L., & Barr, H. M. (2000). On categorizations in analyses of alcohol teratogenesis. *Environmental health perspectives, 108* (Suppl 3), 421–428.

Sampson P. D., Streissguth A. P., Bookstein F. L., Little R. E., Clarren S. K., Dehaene P., et al. (1997). Incidence of fetal alcohol syndrome and prevalence of alcohol-related neurodevelopmental disorder. *Teratology, 56*, 317–326.

Scrimshaw, N. S. (1997). The relation between fetal malnutrition and chronic disease in later life. *BMJ, 315*(7112), 825–826.

Vorhees, C. V., & Mollnow, E. (1987). Behavioral teratogenesis: Long-term influences on behavior from early exposure to environmental agents. In J. D. Osofsky (Ed.), *Wiley Series on Personality Processes. Handbook of Infant Development* (pp. 913–971). Oxford, England: John Wiley & Sons.

Yates, W. R., et al. (1998). Effect of fetal alcohol exposure on adult symptoms of nicotine, alcohol, and drug dependence. *Alcoholism: Clinical and Experimental Research, 22*(4), 914–920.

3. ESSENTIALS OF PSYCHIATRIC EVALUATION OF CHILDREN AND ADOLESCENTS

OBJECTIVES

This chapter will outline essential concepts of psychiatric evaluation, special considerations in evaluating children, the purpose of the interview, components of psychiatric evaluation, interview techniques, steps of an evaluation, mental-status examination, diagnosis, and management.

ESSENTIAL CONCEPTS

Providing a comprehensive initial psychiatric evaluation is the cornerstone of effective treatment planning. The psychiatric evaluation is typically initiated with adults and engaging the child is essential. A comprehensive evaluation includes gathering information from multiple sources, e.g., parents, guardians, child, school, and others. Strengths and deficits need to be identified. The assessment of parent and family functioning is integral to the evaluation.

The purpose of the interview is to:

1) Obtain historical perspective of the patient's life
2) Establish rapport and therapeutic alliance
3) Understand present functioning

4) Make diagnosis
5) Establish a treatment plan

SPECIAL CONSIDERATIONS IN EVALUATING CHILDREN

The psychiatric evaluation of a child or adolescent has a number of important differences from that of an adult:

- The referral is typically requested by someone other than the patient.
- The child may feel ashamed, angry, or convinced the evaluation is a punishment for being "bad."
- Try to set the stage to be as non-critical and nonjudgmental as possible, giving the child as much control as is appropriate as long as they are safe.
- They are not "little adults" (remember the developmental stages). They still need adult supervision and care.
- Use multiple informants: It is important to know if the child is having difficulties in all contexts or only in specific contexts. For example, is the child doing well at school but having behavioural problems at home? This may help clarify the nature of the difficulty and point to specific areas for remediation.
- Diagnosis is more complicated in children. The varying presentation of symptoms at different ages, evolution of disorders, and the lack of diagnostic and etiological specificity for many symptoms make diagnosis more fluid and unclear.
- Different methods of collecting data and interviewing the child apply at different ages. The goal is to understand the child's inner world and perspective.

- The techniques may range from observing an infant-parent dyad, to using play to understand the preschool and young elementary school child, to talking directly about symptoms with the adolescent.
- It should be clarified that the diagnosis may change over time. However, this should not delay the intervention and treatment of disabling symptoms.
- The assessment of parental and family functioning is crucial. It is not possible to conduct an adequate assessment without an understanding of family relationships and the child's response to them. It is important to explore environmental characteristics as well.

COMPONENTS OF A THOROUGH PSYCHIATRIC EVALUATION

Referral source: Who is requesting the assessment and for what purpose? Incorporate information from multiple informants.

Chief complaints and goal of the assessments: What are the difficulties that prompted the evaluation? Find out in what contexts problems occur.

Family evaluation: See the entire family together whenever possible.

INTERVIEW TECHNIQUES

Arrange a comfortable setting with privacy.

Introduce yourself.

Explain the purpose of the interview.

Put the patient at ease, establish a rapport, show empathy.

Do not make value judgments.

Carefully observe patient's nonverbal behaviour, posture, mannerisms, and physical appearance.

Keep the interview active.

Do not argue or get angry.

Use language that is compatible with patient's intelligence.

PSYCHIATRIC INTERVIEW

The psychiatric interview has two parts:

1. The history-taking
2. The mental-status examination

Psychiatric history: The chronological story of the patient's life from birth to present

Mental status: A cross-section of the patient's psychological life. It represents the interviewer's observation and impression at the moment and can be used as a source of referral and a source of information if the patient cannot cooperate. It also serves as a future comparison as the progress of the patient is followed.

Identifying data: Name, age, sex, race, marital status, religion, education, address, occupation

Chief complaints: Brief statement in the patient's own words as to why the patient is in hospital or being seen in consultation

History of present illness: Development of symptoms from time of onset to present, relationship of the events, and change from previous level of functioning

Review other psychiatric symptoms: Rule out comorbidity

Psychosocial stressors: Home, school, friends

Medication history: Current medication, past and present psychotropic medication use

Allergies

History of drugs and alcohol abuse

Previous psychiatric history, hospitalization, outpatient treatment, attempted suicide or self-injurious behaviour

Past medical illness: Neurological illness, surgery

FAMILY HISTORY

Family constellation

Parental employment

Parental psychiatric illness or genetically related family members

Parental legal problems, substance abuse

Parental medical illness

Child and family strengths and weaknesses

Age, gender, and emotional/behavioural problems of other siblings

PREGNANCY, BIRTH AND DEVELOPMENTAL MILESTONES

Pregnancy: Including any medications, use of illicit substances, major illness, or complications

Birth history: Any complication during delivery and early infancy including temperament

Developmental milestones: Including walking, talking, feeding, and toilet training

Educational history: From preschool onwards, including any special services or special education

Peer relationships, activities

Electronics: Use of internet, video games, TV, movies. How much and what types?

Cultural context: Migration history, ethnic identifications, religious affiliations, etc.

Trauma history: Physical or sexual abuse, neglect, witnessing violence, and level of psychosocial adversity

Substance use

Legal history and risk-taking behaviour

Sexual behaviour

MENTAL-STATUS EXAMINATION

General appearance: note appearance, gait, dress, grooming, posture, gestures, facial expression (anxious, tense, panicky, bewildered, sad, unhappy)

Motoric behaviour: psychomotor agitation or retardation, tremor, grimacing, eye contact

Voice: faint, loud, hoarse

Attitude during interview (how patient relates to you): irritable, aggressive, seductive, guarded, defensive, apathetic, cooperative, sarcastic

Mood: steady or sustained emotional state, gloomy, tense, hopeless, resentful, happy, sad, elated, euphoric, depressed, apathetic, anhedonic, fearful, suicidal, grandiose, nihilistic

Affect: state of emotional tone or feeling and may vary from elation, labile, blunt or depression

Speech: slow, fast, pressured, spontaneous, stammering, slurring, aphasia, coprolalia, echolalia, incoherent, mute

THOUGHT PROCESS

Goal-directed ideas

Loosened association

Illogical

Tangential

Relevant

Circumstantial

Rambling ability to abstract

Flight of ideas

Clang association

Perseveration

THOUGHT CONTENT

Delusions (false belief):

- Persecutory delusions (paranoia)
- Delusions of grandeur
- Delusions of guilt
- Hypochondriacal delusions
- Nihilistic delusions
- Religious delusions
- Delusions of influence

Thought broadcasting and insertion

Ideas of reference

Thought blocking

Phobias

Obsession

Assessment of risk: suicidal preoccupation, impulsivity, planning, ability to follow through and means to carry out a plan

Homicidal thoughts or plan

PERCEPTUAL DISTURBANCE

Auditory hallucination

Visual hallucination

Olfactory hallucination

Tactile hallucination

Gustatory hallucination

Hypnopompic hallucination

Hypnagogic hallucination

SENSORIUM (LEVEL OF CONSCIOUSNESS)

Alert

Clear

Confused: a state of disordered orientation

Clouded: impairment of perception, orientation, and attention

Stuporous: semi-comatose stage

Comatose: almost all consciousness is lost, no voluntary activity

Orientation: awareness of one's physical relationship to reality, e.g., time, place, and person

COGNITIVE FUNCTION

Concentration and calculation: Subtract 7 from 100 and keep subtracting (e.g., 100, 93, 86, ...)

Immediate memory: Ask 6 digits forward then backward. Ask to remember three unrelated words and test them after 5 minutes.

Recent memory: Where were you yesterday?

Long-term memory: Where were you born?

Information and intelligence: Who is the president of the United States? Name the capital of Vietnam.

MINI MENTAL-STATE EXAM

Orientation and registration: name of three objects

Attention and calculation: subtract 7 from 100 in serial fashion

Recall three objects

Language test: naming pen, watch

Comprehension: pick up the paper in your right hand, fold it, and place on the floor, read and perform the command; "close your eyes" and write any sentence

Construction: copy the design below

Clinical estimates of cognitive skills and development

Maximum score of mini-mental-state exam = 30

JUDGMENT AND INSIGHT

Judgment: Ability to understand the relationship between facts and to draw conclusions

Response in a social situation

Insight level: Realizing that there is a physical or mental problem

Denial of illness

Blaming outside factors

Recognizing the need for treatment

FORMULATION

Formulation involves a brief statement of the clinician's understanding of the patient's emotional/behavioural problem. It includes the significant findings with an explanation, leading to a diagnosis and a feasible plan for management.

It is suggested that the formulation might be brought together under the following headings:

- A brief outline of the presenting problems and history of the present illness
- Review of predisposing, precipitating factors that account for illness
- A brief synopsis of the relevant findings (positive or negative) in the mental status
- Diagnosis: differential diagnosis if appropriate
- Etiology
- Management plan
- Possible outcome

DIAGNOSIS

The 5-axial DSM-IV diagnostic system has been removed from DSM-V in favour of non-axial documentation of diagnosis for children and adults.

This new approach will combine the former axes I, II and III with separate notations for psychosocial factors (formerly Axis IV) and disability (formerly Axis V).

The dimensional diagnostic system better correlates with treatment planning and medical and neurologic examination.

Differential diagnosis

Prognosis

Treatment plan

INVESTIGATION PROPOSED

Medical evaluation: Obtain the medical history and complete the physical examination, preferably by a pediatrician.

If there is a need for a neurological assessment, it may require one from a pediatric neurologist.

Clarify if any further laboratory workup is needed, including invasive and non-invasive tests.

Psychoeducational testing: to rule out learning disability and intellectual impairments.

Psychological testing to assess executive functioning and projective testing.

Speech and language assessments.

A classroom observation may be helpful.

Rating scales: Vanderbilt and Conners for ADHD, Beck inventory for depression, etc. to assess the severity of symptoms. Baseline and follow up rating scales are helpful in monitoring.

School functioning: communication with teachers is helpful in understanding difficulties and strengths.

MANAGEMENT

Medication management, including psychostimulants, antidepressants, antipsychotics, mood stabilizers, benzodiazepine, and others

Psychological management, including individual, group, and family therapy

Psychosocial intervention: classroom strategy, case management, etc.

Prognosis for present episode

Prognosis for long-term management

CONCLUSION

A comprehensive psychiatric evaluation is the cornerstone of effective treatment planning. A biopsychosocial assessment of the child involving the caregiver would be the most effective approach.

REFERENCES

Lyttle, J. (1986). Mental disorder: Its care and treatment. London, United Kingdom: Bailliere Tindall.

Sadock, B. J. (2003). *Kaplan & Sadock's Synopsis of Psychiatry* (9th ed.). B. J. Sadock & V. A. Sadock (Eds.). Philadelphia, Pennsylvania, United States: Lippincott Williams & Wilkins.

Stubbe, D. (2007). *Child and Adolescent Psychiatry*. Philadelphia, Pennsylvania, United States: Lippincott Williams & Wilkins.

4. INTELLECTUAL DISABILITY

OBJECTIVES

This chapter will discuss the definition, epidemiology, causes, and symptoms of intellectual disability (ID). Assessment, management, and long-term outcomes of IDs will be discussed as well.

DEFINITION

Intellectual disability (ID) is a term that describes individuals whose intelligence (thinking, reasoning, problem-solving abilities) and daily-living skills are well below other people of the same age. Other terms for ID are developmental disability (DD) and mental retardation. When a child is very young, terms like developmental delay or global developmental delay may be used. Some of these children may later be diagnosed with ID.

EPIDEMIOLOGY

The global Disease Control Priorities Project (DCPP) estimates that 10% to 20% of individuals worldwide have a developmental disability of some kind. In the US alone, it is estimated that 9% of children younger than 36 months of age have a possible developmental problem, while 13.87% of children 3–17 years of age have a developmental disability.

CAUSES OF INTELLECTUAL DISABILITY

Trauma before birth, such as infection or exposure to alcohol, drugs, or other toxins

Trauma during birth, such as oxygen deprivation or premature delivery

Chromosome abnormalities, such as Down syndrome

Severe malnutrition or other dietary issues

Severe cases of early childhood illness, such as whooping cough, measles, or meningitis

Brain injury

SYMPTOMS OF INTELLECTUAL DISABILITY

Symptoms of ID will vary based on the child's level of disability and may include:

- Failure to meet intellectual milestones
- Sitting, crawling, or walking later than other children
- Problems learning to talk or difficulty speaking clearly
- Memory problems
- Inability to understand the consequences of actions
- Inability to think logically
- Childish behaviour inconsistent with the child's age
- Lack of curiosity
- Learning difficulties
- IQ below 70
- Inability to lead a fully independent life due to challenges

If a child has ID, they may experience some of the following behavioural issues:

- Aggression
- Dependency
- Withdrawal from social activities
- Attention-seeking behaviour
- Depression during adolescent and teen years
- Lack of impulse control
- Passivity
- Tendency towards self-injury
- Stubbornness
- Low self-esteem
- Low tolerance for frustration
- Psychotic disorders
- Difficulty paying attention

LEVELS OF INTELLECTUAL DISABILITY

ID is divided into four levels, based on a child's IQ and degree of social adjustment:

1) Mild Intellectual Disability

Symptoms include:
- Taking longer to learn to talk, but communicating well once they know how to
- Being fully independent in self-care when they get older
- Having problems with reading and writing
- Social immaturity

- Benefitting from specialized education plans
- Having an IQ range of 50 to 69

2) Moderate Intellectual Disability

Symptoms include:
- Slow in understanding and using language
- May have some difficulties with communication
- Can learn basic reading, writing, and counting skills
- Are generally unable to live alone
- Can often get around on their own to familiar places
- Can take part in various types of social activities
- Generally having an IQ range of 35 to 49

3) Severe Intellectual Disability

Symptoms include:
- Noticeable motor impairment
- Severe damage to, or abnormal development of, their central nervous system
- Generally having an IQ range of 20 to 34

4) Profound Intellectual Disability

Symptoms include:
- Inability to understand or comply with requests or instructions
- Possible immobility
- Incontinence
- Need for constant help and supervision
- Having an IQ of less than 20

ASSESSMENT

Interview with parents

Observation of the child

Standard tests

The evaluation process usually includes a psychologist, pediatric neurologist, developmental pediatrician, and physical therapist.

The child will be given standard intelligence tests, such as the Stanford-Binet intelligence test to determine the child's IQ.

The Vineland Adaptive Behavior Scale provides an assessment of daily-living skills and social abilities compared to other children in the same age group.

It is important to remember that children from different cultures and socioeconomic statuses may perform differently on these tests.

Laboratory and imaging tests may also be performed to detect structural problems with the child's brain, as well as metabolic and genetic disorders.

Other conditions, such as hearing loss, learning disorders, neurological disorders, and emotional problems can also cause delayed development.

TREATMENT OPTIONS FOR INTELLECTUAL DISABILITY

The main goal of treatment is to help the child reach his/her full potential in terms of:

- Education
- Social skills
- Life skills

Treatment may include:

- Individualized education program (IEP)
- Speech therapy
- Physiotherapy
- Behavioural therapy
- Occupational therapy
- Counselling
- Medication, in some cases
- Family support

LONG-TERM OUTCOME

If ID occurs with other serious physical problems, the child may have a below-average life expectancy.

If the child has mild to moderate ID, they will probably have a fairly normal life expectancy.

If support services are available, a child growing up with mild ID may live an independent and fulfilling life as an adult.

CONCLUSION

A child with an intellectual disability (ID) will have thinking, reasoning, and problem-solving skills below other children of the same age. Prevalence rate: fairly common. Causes are biological or environmental and timing of exposure (before, during, after birth).

There are different levels of intellectual disability. Symptoms of ID vary based on levels of disability. ID is formally diagnosed through a multidisciplinary approach. The child needs biopsychosocial support to thrive well, and with favourable support and depending on the level of disability may live independently as an adult.

ONLINE RESOURCES

aaid.org (American Association on Intellectual and Developmental Disabilities)

communityinclusion.org (Answers to parents' questions on mental retardation)

cacl.ca (Canadian Association for Community Living)

ctnsy.ca (Children's Treatment Network of Simcoe York; Intellectual disabilities: an introduction for families)

kidshealth.org (Kids Health)

kidsnewtocanada.ca/mental-health/prenatal-risk (Prenatal risk factors for developmental delay in newcomer children; (July 2019) Canadian Paediatric Society)

healthline.com/health/developmental-delay (What you should know about developmental delay)

healthline.com/health/mental-retardation (What you should know about intellectual disability)

5. THE AUTISM SPECTRUM DISORDERS

OBJECTIVE

This chapter will discuss the DSM-5 diagnostic criteria for autism spectrum disorder (ASD) and social (pragmatic) communication disorder. The epidemiology, developmental warning signs, characteristic features, differential diagnosis, comorbidities, evaluation, and management of ASDs will be discussed.

INTRODUCTION

Autism spectrum disorder (ASD) is a neurodevelopmental disorder, presenting the core features of abnormal relatedness and social development. Cognitive and motor development is also affected.

DSM-5 DIAGNOSTIC CRITERIA OF AUTISM SPECTRUM DISORDER

A) Persistent deficits in social communication and social interaction across multiple contexts as follows:
- Deficits in social and emotional reciprocity
- Deficits in nonverbal communicative behaviours
- Deficits in developing, maintaining, and understanding relationships

B) Restricted, repetitive patterns of behaviour, interests, or activities manifested by at least two of the following:

- Stereotype or repetitive motor movements
- Insistence on sameness, inflexible adherence to routine, or ritualistic patterns of verbal or nonverbal behaviours
- Highly restricted, fixed interest in unusual objects
- Hyper- or hypo-reactivity to sensory input, e.g., pain, temperature, texture of food or clothing, excessive smelling or touching objects

C) Symptoms must be present in the early developmental period.

D) Symptoms cause clinically significant impairment in social, occupational, or other important areas of current functioning.

E) These disturbances cannot be explained by intellectual disability or global developmental delay.

DSM-5 DIAGNOSTIC CRITERIA OF SOCIAL (PRAGMATIC) COMMUNICATION DISORDER

A) Persistent difficulties in the social use of verbal and nonverbal communication as manifested by all of the following:

- Deficits in using communication for social purposes, e.g., greeting or sharing information
- Impairment of the ability to change communication to match the context or the need of the listener
- Difficulties following rules for conversation, e.g., taking turns in conversation
- Difficulties understanding what is not explicitly stated

B) The deficits result in functional limitations in effective communications, social participation, social relationships, academic achievement or occupational performance.

C) The onset of the symptoms is in the early developmental period.

D) The symptoms are not attributable to other medical or neurological conditions, e.g., ASD, intellectual disability, or other mental illness.

EPIDEMIOLOGY OF ASD

Number of children diagnosed with ASD has increased rapidly in the last 10 years

Approximately 0.1% of the population may have a diagnosable ASD

Prevalence: 2–15 per 10,000

Male to female ratios of 4:1, but girls generally present with a more severe disorder

ASDs present in equal prevalence across race, ethnicity, and nationality

ETIOLOGY OF ASDS

Hereditary: multiple genes involved

Fifty times more prevalent in siblings

High concordance (60% to 90%) in monozygotic twins

Early alterations in embryonic development: prenatal damage to infection, toxins.

Neuroimaging findings: ventricular enlargement, larger brain.

Neurotransmitter abnormalities: abnormalities in glutamate, serotonin, dopamine, and GABA neurotransmitters

DEVELOPMENTAL WARNING SIGNS OF ASD

Preschool children:

- Delay or absence of spoken language
- Looks through people, not aware of others
- Not responsive to other people's facial expressions/feelings
- Lack of pretend play, little or no imagination
- Does not show typical interest in or play near peers, purposeful lack of turn-taking
- Unable to share pleasure
- Impairment of nonverbal communication
- Does not point at an object to direct another person to look at it
- Lack of gaze monitoring
- Lack of initiating of activity or social play
- Unusual or repetitive hand or finger mannerisms
- Unusual reactions or lack of reaction to sensory stimuli

School-age children—communication impairment:

- Abnormalities in language development
- Odd or inappropriate prosody (patterns of rhythm and sound)
- Persistent echolalia
- Reference to self as "you," "she," or "he" beyond 3 years
- Unusual vocabulary for child's age/social group
- Limited use of language for communication
- Tendency to talk freely only about specific topics

School-age children—social impairment:

- Inability to join in play of other children or inappropriate attempts at joint play (may manifest as aggressive or disruptive behaviour)
- Lack of awareness of classroom "norms"
- Easily overwhelmed by social or other situations
- Failure to relate normally to adults
- Shows extreme reactions to invasion of personal space and resistant to being hurried

School-age children—impairments of interest, activities, and behaviours:

- Lack of flexible cooperative imaginative play/creativity
- Difficulty in organizing self in relation to unstructured space
- Inability to cope with change or unstructured situation, even ones that other children enjoy (school trip, teacher being away, etc.)
- Other factors: unusual profile of skills/deficits, any other evidence of odd behaviours including unusual responses to sensory stimuli

CLINICAL COURSE OF ASD

Lifelong course, language skills, and overall IQ are strongest prognostic indicators

Mental retardation common and 0.25% have seizures in adolescence

DIFFERENTIAL DIAGNOSIS OF AUTISM SPECTRUM DISORDER

Selective mutism: child is able to speak and does so with family

Developmental language disorders: may use nonverbal cues, generally well-related

Reactive attachment disorder: history of severe abuse/neglect

COMORBID MENTAL DISORDERS

Comorbidity is common with ASD. Approximately 80% of children have associated mental retardation, anxiety disorders, commonly obsessive-compulsive disorder and attention deficit hyperactivity disorder (ADHD). Tic disorders, psychotic symptoms, and learning disorders are also common.

EVALUATION FOR CHILDREN WITH ASD (CLINICAL HISTORY)

Focus on prenatal and perinatal history and early language and social development

Sensory sensitivities to sound, light, tactile, and olfactory stimulation

Odd or repetitive behaviours

Ability to make transitions or change in routine

Family history

Medical history

Focus on eye contact, ability to relate, ability for reciprocal and imaginative play or talk

Note perseveration on a topic or activity, tone of voice and intonation, delayed or unusual speech

Need for doing things in a particular manner or to be in charge of how things are done in a persistent and intense manner

Observation of child's functioning in school or at home may also be helpful

Medical and neurological assessment and hearing test

Psychological testing to determine cognitive level, adaptive functioning and mental retardation

Academic testing to rule out learning disabilities

Young children should have a developmental evaluation

Miscellaneous: Speech and language testing, occupational- and physical-therapy evaluation

MANAGEMENT OF ASD

General principles of ASD management:

- ASDs can present substantial barriers to normal daily functioning
- Approach to its management is a combination of symptom modification together with the removal of these barriers wherever possible
- Address co-existing conditions to manage the core ASD symptoms

Non-pharmacological management:

- Parent-delivered and clinician-delivered interventions which include:
    - Communication intervention: wide range of methods and techniques designed to improve communication, including social and nonverbal communication. Often this work is conducted by speech and language therapists.
    - Social-skills intervention: Designed to encourage more effective interpersonal interactions, such as social communication therapy, tactile promoting, and visual reinforcement.

Educational approach:

- These include both entire behavioural programs and specific interventions for problems ranging from self-harming behaviours to difficulties in sleep
- Applied behavioural analysis (ABA): plan that teaches appropriate behaviours that are to be generalized to all domains of child's environment
- Social stories: the use of stories to problem-solve social dilemmas
- Discrete trial training (DTT): teaching skills in specific situations
- Developmental individual difference relationship model (DIR): uses relationship method to help the child relate and attend to the social setting
- Treatment and education of autistic and handicapped children: collaboration between mental health and education professionals with parents to formulate an effective education and treatment plan

Psychosocial approach:

- Family support: individual support, counselling, support group
- Parent psycho-education: teaching parents about the disorder and collaboration in treatment planning
- Parent behavioural management training: use of a behavioural specialist to help parents learn to employ behavioural management protocols to help their child learn appropriate behaviour
- Public education system: special education services individualized to the need of the child

- Referral for special therapies: speech therapies for delay and to teach social speech; occupational therapy for sensory processing and fine motor deficits; physiotherapy for coordination deficits
- Referral for disability services and support: ensure that child and family gain appropriate entitlements and supports with the child and family's needs

Psychopharmacological intervention:

- Antipsychotics: risperidone, aripiprazole, olanzapine, quetiapine, ziprasidone, haloperidol
    - Target symptoms: Aggression, agitation, irritability, hyperactivity, and self-injurious behaviour
    - Comments: These medications are used to treat behavioural disturbances in ASD. Most common adverse effects are weight gain, hyperlipidemia, hypertension, and increased prolactin.
- Selective serotonin reuptake inhibitors (SSRIs): fluoxetine, sertraline, escitalopram, citalopram, fluvoxamine, venlafaxine (serotonin-noradrenaline reuptake inhibitors (SNRI))
    - Target symptoms: Anxiety, perseveration, compulsive behaviour, depression, and social isolation
    - Comments: Positive response may be correlated with a family history of affective disorder. Potential adverse effects are restlessness, insomnia, mania.
- Alfa-2 agonists: clonidine, guanfacine
    - Target symptoms: hyperactivity, aggression, and sleep dysregulation
    - Comments: Clonidine is more sedating.

- Anticonvulsants and lithium:
  ○ Target symptoms: Aggression and self-injurious behaviour. May help mood lability.
  ○ Comments: Need for blood monitoring may limit use.
- Stimulants: methylphenidate, dextroamphetamine compounds
  ○ Target symptoms: Hyperactivity and inattention
  ○ Comments: Variable response. May increase agitation and stereotypic behaviours.

CONCLUSION

The essential features of ASD are abnormal social development and relatedness. Early detection and intervention improve prognosis. Treatment should be multimodal and multidimensional. Anxiety and other psychiatric disorders may complicate prognosis and treatment.

REFERENCES

American Psychiatric Association. (2013). Diagnostic and statistical manual of mental disorders (5th ed.). Arlington, VA, US: American Psychiatric Publishing, Inc.

Coghill, D., Graham, J., & Bonnar, S., et al. (2009). *Child and Adolescent Psychiatry*. Oxford, United Kingdom: Oxford University Press.

Stubbe, D. (2007). *Child and Adolescent Psychiatry*. Philadelphia, Pennsylvania, United States: Lippincott Williams & Wilkins.

6. ATTENTION DEFICIT HYPERACTIVITY DISORDER

OBJECTIVES

This chapter will outline the DSM-5 diagnostic criteria for ADHD. Symptom manifestation across the life, comorbidities, differential diagnosis, biopsychosocial assessment, risk of not treating ADHD, pharmacological and psychosocial intervention including comorbidity, and course and prognosis of ADHD will be covered.

INTRODUCTION

Attention deficit hyperactivity disorder (ADHD) is the most commonly diagnosed behavioural disorder of childhood and adolescence. It is characterized by attention difficulties, hyperactivity and impulsivity.

The onset of symptoms appears at a very young age, and symptoms persist throughout the lifetime with significant comorbidity with other psychiatric disorders.

A multimodal, biopsychosocial approach is taken for treating ADHD. If left untreated, ADHD can lead to more severe disruptive behavioural disorders and can become an economic and social burden.

EPIDEMIOLOGY OF ADHD

Affects 6% to 9% of school-age children

Persistence of ADHD into adolescence is 70%

Persistence of ADHD into adulthood is 50% to 60%

Worldwide prevalence of ADHD is 3% to 7%

Current population estimates of 4.4% rate of ADHD in adults

Male to female ratio in school-age children ranges from 3:1 to 9:1 in clinic referral samples and 2:1 in community-based samples.

CAUSE OF ADHD

ADHD is most likely caused by a complex interplay of the following factors:

- Neuroanatomical/neurochemical
- Genetic origin
- Central Nervous System (CNS) insults
- Environmental factors

DSM-5 DIAGNOSTIC CRITERIA FOR ADHD

Onset of symptoms before 12 years of age.

Symptoms must persist for 6 months.

Impairment must be present in two or more settings.

There must be clear evidence of clinically significant impairment of functioning.

Symptoms are not exclusively due to other medical, neurological, or psychiatric disorders.

Inattention:

- Is careless
- Has difficulty sustaining attention

- Does not listen
- Does not follow through with tasks
- Is disorganized
- Avoids/dislikes tasks requiring sustained effort
- Loses important items
- Is easily distracted
- Is forgetful in daily activities

Hyperactivity:
- Squirms and fidgets
- Cannot stay seated
- Runs/climbs excessively
- Cannot play/work quietly
- Is on the go
- Talks excessively

Impulsivity:
- Blurts out answers
- Cannot wait for turn
- Intrudes/interrupts others

Subtypes:
- Hyperactive/impulsive type: at least six hyperactivity/impulsivity items
- Inattentive type: at least six inattentiveness items
- Combined type: at least six inattentiveness items plus six hyperactivity/impulsivity items

ADHD SYMPTOMS MANIFEST THROUGHOUT LIFE

Preschool: Behavioural disturbance

School Age: Behavioural disturbance, academic problems, difficulty with social interactions, self-esteem issues

Adolescence: Academic problems, difficulty with social interactions, self-esteem issues, legal issues, smoking and injury

College Age: Academic failure, occupational difficulties, self-esteem issues, substance abuse, injury/accidents

Adult: Occupational failure, self-esteem issues, relationship problems, injury/accidents, substance abuse

CHILDHOOD ADHD COMMON CO-MORBIDITIES

Oppositional Defiant Disorder (ODD)

Conduct disorder

Tics

Obsessive-Compulsive Disorder (OCD)

Learning disorders

Substance-use disorders

Anxiety disorders

Mood disorders

ADHD DIAGNOSTIC ASSESSMENT TECHNIQUES

Interview → History → Standardized assessment measures → Physical and neurological examination

ADHD DIFFERENTIAL DIAGNOSIS

Environmental:
- Abuse or neglect

- Family adversity

Medical:
- Absence seizures
- Sensory deficits
- Thyroid disorders

Neurodevelopmental:
- Learning disorder
- Speech and language disorder
- Social (pragmatic) communication disorder, autism spectrum disorders (ASDs)

Psychiatric:
- Conduct disorder
- Oppositional defiant disorder (ODD)
- Anxiety disorder
- Mood disorder
- Substance-abuse disorder

RISKS OF NOT TREATING CHILD AND ADOLESCENT ADHD

Increased risk of tobacco smoking

Increased risk of alcohol/substance abuse

Increased risk of pregnancy in girls

Increased risk of driving accidents

Increased risk of dropping out of school

Increased risk of frequent job changes

ADHD TREATMENT CHOICES

For severe, pervasive, and disabling ADHD: Medication + psychosocial management

Otherwise:

- For school-based problems: Teacher and classroom modification
- For home-based problems: Parent training and behavioural intervention in the family
- For persistent symptoms and impairment after psychosocial management: Medication + psychosocial management

ADHD PHARMACOTHERAPY TREATMENT OPTIONS

Stimulants:

Methylphenidate

- Ritalin/Ritalin SR
- Biphentin
- Concerta
- Foquest

Amphetamine compounds

- Dexedrine tablet
- Dexedrine Spansule capsule
- Adderall XR
- Vyvanse

Non-Stimulants:

- Atomoxetine

Antihypertensives:
- Clonidine
- Guanfacine

Antidepressants:
- Bupropion
- Tricyclics

Stimulants are found to improve:
- Core symptoms
- Inattention
- Hyperactivity
- Impulsivity

Others:
- Noncompliance
- Social interactions
- Impulsive aggression
- Academic productivity

ADVANTAGES OF LONG-ACTING STIMULANT FORMULATIONS

For patients experiencing very brief duration of effect from standard formulations.

In situations where frequent dosing is inconvenient, stigmatizing, or impossible (in school dosing).

More consistent and stable plasma levels of drug coverage throughout the day. May improve medication compliance and better parental control. May decrease abuse potential.

AREAS OF CONCERN AND CONTROVERSY WITH STIMULANT USE AND ADVERSE EFFECTS

Dextroamphetamine and methylphenidate have similar side effect profiles:

- Growth suppression
- Medication abuse
- Cardiovascular effects
- Decreased appetite
- Headache
- Stomach upset
- Insomnia
- Irritability
- Anxiety

SIDE-EFFECT MANAGEMENT STRATEGIES

Decreased appetite:

- Monitor weight, give high-calorie snacks/bedtime snacking
- Consider drug holidays

Headaches/stomach aches:

- Decrease dose
- Switch to another stimulant
- Switch to second-line agent

Insomnia:

- Administer dose earlier in the day
- Adjunctive pharmacotherapy
- Avoidance of coffee/tea

RECOMMENDATION FOR STARTING AND MAXIMUM DOSES OF STIMULANTS

Methylphenidate:

- Child: 5 mg am and noon, maximum dose 60 mg/day
- Adolescent: 5 mg am and noon, maximum dose 60 mg/day

Dexedrine:

- Child: 5 mg am and noon, maximum dose 30 mg/day
- Adolescent: 5 mg am and noon, maximum dose 30 mg/day

Concerta:

- Child: 18 mg am, maximum dose 72 mg am
- Adolescent: 18 mg am, maximum dose 72 mg am

Adderall XR:

- Child: 10 mg am, maximum dose 30 mg am
- Adolescent 10 mg am, maximum dose 60 mg am

Biphentin:

- Child: 10 mg am, maximum dose 60 mg am
- Adolescent: 10 mg am, maximum dose 60 mg am

Source: Canadian ADHD Resource Alliance (CADDRA), 2006

Vyvanse (lisdexamfetamine dimesylate):

- Only prodrug for the treatment of ADHD in children and adolescents
- Efficacy within 1.5 hrs and lasts up to 13 hrs post-dose

- Mechanism of action: Lisdexamfetamine is a prodrug of amphetamine. After oral administration, inactive prodrug is rapidly absorbed in the GI tract and converted to active d-amphetamine by natural enzymatic processes.
- Easy dosing once a day available in 10 mg, 20 mg, 30 mg, 40 mg, 50 mg, and 60 mg. Usual dose for starting or switching 10 mg to 20 mg OD am. Maximum dose should not exceed 70 mg OD am.
- Side effects include: Decreased appetite, insomnia, abdominal pain, headache, irritability, vomiting, weight decrease, and nausea.
- Serious side effects include: Slowing of growth, seizures (mainly patient with a history of seizures), eyesight changes or blurred vision warnings, heart disease, structural heart abnormalities, high blood pressure, family history of sudden death, or death related to heart problems

Atomoxetine (selective norepinephrine reuptake inhibitor):
- Indication for atomoxetine:
  - Patient not responsive to stimulants
  - Patients with significant side effects to stimulants, e.g., tics, patients with Tourette's syndrome or chronic motor-tic disorders, comorbid anxiety
  - Abuse or diversion is a concern with stimulants
  - Epilepsy

Problems:
- 6–8 weeks titration
- Slow metabolizers

Side effects:

- Dry mouth
- Insomnia
- Nausea
- Constipation
- Decreased appetite
- Dizziness
- Liver toxicity

PSYCHOSOCIAL TREATMENT OF ADHD

Work with the child:

- Social-skills training: to learn social and academic problem-solving strategies and the ability to manage frustration
- Individual psychotherapy: useful for addressing comorbid disorders, issues of self-esteem or sequelae of trauma

Parent psychoeducation:

- Education about the disorder, teaching how to manage the environment to assist the child
- Consistencies of routine, organization, reducing stimulation, decreasing frustration, anticipating difficulties, and behavioural management

Family therapy:

- To reduce conflict and improve communication and problem solving within the family

Parent training and behavioural intervention in the family:

- Encouraging continual monitoring of child's progress
- Analysis of the positive and negative consequences

- Identification of specific problems and situations leading to disruptive behaviour
- Use of time-out for more serious forms of problem behaviour
- Reduction of coercive and unpleasant parent-child interactions
- Teaching parents effective methods of communicating commands and rule-setting
- Use of token systems to reinforce appropriate behaviour in specific situations
- Identification of marked inconsistencies of applying negative consequences to problem behaviour

Teacher and classroom modifications:
- Discussion of classroom structure and task demands with the teacher
- Having child sit close to the teacher
- Brief academic assignments
- Spacing classroom lectures with brief periods of physical exercise
- Frequent monitoring of the child's progress with a rating scale
- Consistent classroom structure and routine, organizational skills teaching
- Assisting child in organizing notebook, materials, and homework assignments
- Extra supervision in unstructured activities, e.g., lunch, recess
- Use of token system to reinforce positive behaviour
- Use of brief time-out for serious forms of problem behaviour and noncompliance

TREATMENT OF ADHD AND COMORBIDITY

ADHD + ODD and Conduct Disorder (CD):

- Combination of stimulant medication, mood stabilizer, and atypical antipsychotics are effective for ADHD symptoms and to decrease verbal aggression, physical aggression, negative social interaction, covert antisocial behaviour
- Family therapy and behavioural management therapy is helpful
- Efficacy may rely on concurrent medication management

ADHD + Tics and Tourette's

- Can try stimulants; may make ADHD worse
- If stimulants make tics worse, try atomoxetine
- If still problematic, add risperidone

ADHD + Substance Abuse:

- Need to treat ADHD
- Substance-abuse counselling
- Be careful with diversion

ADHD + Anxiety:

- Prioritize treatment: What is most debilitating?
- Combination therapy often required
- Stimulants are first-line therapy for ADHD symptoms
- SSRI antidepressants are effective for anxiety
- Also consider benzodiazepine, buspirone, and atomoxetine

ADHD + Bipolar Disorder:
- Treat bipolar condition first
- Mood stabilizers: lithium, valproate
- Atypical antipsychotics
- Once mood becomes stable, add stimulants

ADHD + Depression:
- If severe, treat depression prior to ADHD
- Consider SSRIs + stimulants, bupropion

ADHD + ASD:
- Try atypical antipsychotics, risperidone, quetiapine, aripiprazole
- Can try stimulants; may not be that effective

COURSE AND PROGNOSIS OF ADHD

About three-quarters of children diagnosed with ADHD continue to show symptoms of ADHD into adolescence. Persistence of ADHD into adulthood is 50% to 60%. Risk factors determining the persistence of ADHD diagnosis in adults are associated with increased severity of ADHD symptoms, presence of comorbidities, adversities during childhood, and family history of ADHD.

About one-third of ADHD children show features of conduct disorder. Children with ADHD and CD are at higher risk for developing substance-use disorders and antisocial personality in adulthood.

ADHD children often show low self-esteem and poor social skills. One-third of ADHD children drop out of high school with lower occupational rankings, more car accidents, court appearances and convictions, suicide attempts, and problems with relationships.

Prognosis improves with effective treatment, appropriate educational programming, high cognitive, athletic, and interpersonal abilities, and an emotionally supportive family with adequate social and financial resources.

CONCLUSION

ADHD is caused by a complex interplay of factors such as neuroanatomical, neurochemical, genetic, environmental conditions, and CNS insults. The onset of symptoms appears at a very young age and persists throughout life. It is often associated with significant comorbidity with other psychiatric disorders. A comprehensive diagnostic assessment is needed to clarify diagnosis and comorbidity. A multimodal biopsychosocial approach is taken for treating ADHD. In recent years, several extended-release stimulant and non-stimulant medications have brought about a revolution in the management and treatment of ADHD.

REFERENCES

Adler, L. & Cohen, J. (2004). Diagnosis and evaluation of adults with attention-deficit/hyperactivity disorder. *Psychiatr Clin North Am., 27*(2), 187–201.

American Psychiatric Association. (2013). Diagnostic and statistical manual of mental disorders (5th ed.). Arlington, VA, US: American Psychiatric Publishing, Inc.

Barkey, R. A. (2006). Attention–Deficit Hyperactivity Disorder: A Handbook for Diagnosis And Treatment, Third Edition. New York: The Guilford Press.

Baumgaertel, A., Wolraich, M. L., & Dietrich, M. (1995). Comparison of diagnostic criteria for attention deficit disorders in a German elementary school sample. *J Am Acad Child Adolesc Psychiatry, 34*, 629–638.

Biederman, J., Wilens, T., Mick, E., Faraone, S. V., Weber, W., Curtis, S., et al. (1997). Is ADHD a risk factor for psychoactive substance use disorders? Findings from a four-year prospective follow-up study. *Journal of the American Academy of Child and Adolescent Psychiatry, 36*, 21–29.

Castellanos, F. X. (1999). Stimulants and tic disorders: from dogma to data. *Arch Gen Psychiatry, 56*, 337–338.

Coghill, D., Graham, J., Bonnar, S., et al. (2009). Child and Adolescent Psychiatry. Oxford, United Kingdom: Oxford University Press.

Conners, K. C. & Jett, J. L. (1999). Attention Deficit Hyperactivity Disorder (in Adults and Children): The Latest Assessment and Treatment Strategies. Michigan, USA: Compact Clinicals.

Dulcan, M. (1997). Practice Parameters for the Assessment and Treatment of Children, Adolescents, and Adults With Attention-Deficit/Hyperactivity Disorder. *Journal of the*

American Academy of Child and Adolescent Psychiatry, 36(10), 85S–121S.

Findling, R. L. & Dogin, J. W. (1998). Psychopharmacology of children with ADHD: children and adolescents. *Journal of Clinical Psychiatry, 59* (suppl 7), 42–49.

Goldman, L. S., Genel, M., Bezman, R. J., & Slanetz, P. J. (1998). Diagnosis and treatment of attention-deficit/hyperactivity disorder in children and adolescents. *JAMA, 279*(14), 1100–1107.

Goodman, D. W. (2009). ADHD in adults: update for clinicians on diagnosis and assessment. *Primary Psychiatry, 16*(11) epub.

Kessler, R. C., Adler, L., Barkley, R., et al. (2006). The prevalence & correlates of Adult ADHD in the United States: Results from the national comorbidity survey. *Replication American Journal of Psychiatry, 163*(4), 716–723.

Milberger, S., Biederman, J., Faraone, S. V., Murphy, J., & Tsuang, M. T. (1995). Attention deficit hyperactivity disorder and comorbid disorders: issues of overlapping symptoms. *Am J Psychiatry, 152*(12), 1793–1799.

Petitclere, A. & Tremblay, R. E. (2009). Childhood disruptive behaviour disorders: review of their origin, development, and prevention. *The Canadian Journal of Psychiatry, 54*(4), 222–231.

Pliszka, S. R. (1998). Comorbidity of attention-deficit/hyperactivity disorder with psychiatric disorder: an overview. *J Clin Psychiatry, 59* Suppl 7, 50–58.

Spencer, T. J., Biederman, J., Harding, M., et al. (1996). Growth deficits in ADHD children revisited: evidence for disorder-associated growth delays? *J Am Acad Child Adolesc Psychiatry, 35*, 1460–1469.

Stubbe, D. (2007). *Child and Adolescent Psychiatry*. Philadelphia, Pennsylvania, United States: Lippincott Williams & Wilkins.

Swanson, J. (2003). Compliance with stimulants for attention-deficit/hyperactivity disorder: issues and approaches for improvement. *CNS Drugs, 17*(2), 117–131.

Szatmari, P., Offord, D. R., & Boyle, M. H. (1989). Ontario child health study: Prevalence of attention deficit disorder with hyperactivity. *Journal of Child Psychology and Psychiatry, 30*, 219–230.

Wender, P. H., Wolfe, L. E., & Wasserstein, J. (2006). Adults with ADHD: An Overview. *Annals of the New York Academy of Science, 93*(1), 1–16.

Wolraich, M. L., Hannah, J. N., Baumgaertel, A., et al. (1998). Examination of DSM-IV criteria for attention-deficit/hyperactivity disorder in a county-wide sample. *J Dev Behav Pediatr., 19*, 162–168.

7. OPPOSITIONAL DEFIANT DISORDER

OBJECTIVES

This chapter will outline the characteristics of the inflexible, explosive child (oppositional defiant disorder (ODD)), as well as the epidemiology, etiology, DSM-5 diagnostic criteria, differential diagnosis, and comorbidity of ODD. The dynamics of ODD in terms of the child and the parents' perspective, American Academy of Child and Adolescent Psychiatry (AACAP) guidelines for assessment and treatment of ODD, and the natural course and prevention of ODD will also be discussed.

INTRODUCTION

Oppositional defiant disorder (inflexible, explosive child) is a common, complex, relatively persistent, and potentially disabling condition. More research is needed to describe, understand and better manage ODD. Nonetheless, there are some helpful intervention strategies, many with some research base, which can be utilized.

CHARACTERISTICS OF THE INFLEXIBLE-EXPLOSIVE CHILD

The essential features include:

- Recurrent pattern of negativistic, defiant, hostile, and disobedient behaviour towards authority figures
- Difficulty managing frustration and resolving frustrating situations
- Extremely low frustration threshold; limited capacity for flexibility/adaptability
- Concrete, rigid, black-and-white thinking
- Decreased ability to verbalize emotions

SOME OBSERVATIONS

Despite prevalence and importance, it is a highly neglected area in training and research. In consultative child psychiatry, children and adolescents who are high on the ODD spectrum are very common referrals and amongst the most challenging children for parents, helpers, and the system. There is a tendency to lump disruptive behavioural disorders together. Apart from the high comorbidity, ADHD, ODD, and CD have substantial differences.

ADDITIONAL OBSERVATIONS

Children often have a poor work ethic

Can be self-centred/materialistic/grandiose

Often see the world as treating them unfairly

Often poor at commencing and maintaining interest in activities, sports, etc.

Rarely recognize the extent to which they make life more difficult for their teachers, their families or even themselves

Rarely enthusiastic "customers" for mental health intervention

EPIDEMIOLOGY

ODD may be developmentally normal in early childhood. ODD behaviour can begin as early as 3 years of age. It typically begins by 8 years of age and usually not later than adolescence. Approximately 6% of children are estimated to have ODD. However, prevalence is 5% to 15%. Other groups claim the prevalence is really between 16% and 22%. ODD is more prevalent in boys than in girls before puberty; the sex ratio is probably equal after puberty.

ETIOLOGY

ODD appears to be more common in families where at least one parent has a history of ADHD, CD, mood disorder, antisocial personality disorder or substance-related disorder. Lack of parental supervision, parental unavailability, lack of positive parental involvement, inconsistency in discipline practices, structuring, and limit setting, as well as outright child abuse has been implicated in the pathogenesis of disruptive behaviour. The child may identify with an impulse disordered parent who role models oppositional and defiant interactions with others.

DIAGNOSTIC CRITERIA OF ODD (DSM-5)

Pattern of 1) angry 2) argumentative, and 3) vindictive, lasting at least six months as evidence by at least **four** symptoms from any of the following categories:

1) Angry/ irritable mood

Often loses temper

Often touchy or easily annoyed

Often angry and resentful

2) Argumentative/defiant behaviour

Often argues with authority figures

Often actively defies or refuses to comply

Often deliberately annoys others

Often blames others for his or her mistakes/behaviour

3) Vindictiveness

At least twice in the past month

SOME PROBLEMS WITH ODD DIAGNOSIS

Variability in presentation across time and setting

Need for behavioural questionnaire, e.g., SNAP

Tendency of parents to view ODD as "within child" and overlook interactional contribution

Assumption that with a psychiatric diagnosis we should be able to "fix" child via medication and "talk therapy," etc.

Parental concern regarding labelling, child's reputation

DIFFERENTIAL DIAGNOSIS

Developmental stage

Attention deficit hyperactivity disorder

Adjustment disorder

Mental retardation

Learning disorder

Conduct disorder

Mood and anxiety disorder

COMORBIDITY

ADHD

Conduct disorder

Substance abuse

DYNAMICS OF ODD

Behavioural Perspectives:

- Oppositional and defiant behaviours may be shaped or maintained by ineffective parenting or behavioural strategies, such as:
  - Inconsistent expectations, supervision or discipline by an important caregiver
  - Inconsistencies among caregivers
  - Caregiver lacking in clarity or confidence in their authority role

Family perspectives:

- Oppositional and defiant behaviours are an interactional phenomenon, not within child
- Some children are primarily "oppositional" appearing to go out of their way to provoke and attract negative attention
- Others are primarily "defiant," oriented around doing as they please regardless of rules and expectations
- Some children show a mixture of both features
- Children view themselves as "little adults"
- They view interaction with adults as "win/lose" and are out to show "superiority" over adults
- Their actions are oriented more toward process than content. They have "won" if they "push your buttons" or see you "lose your cool" even if the outcome is negative

- Draw energy off an adult's uncertain, dramatic or frustrated response
- Essentially, they question the competence of adults
- Their behaviours can bring out problematic adult responses, thereby "proving" adult incompetence
- In their drive to be adult-like, these kids may be growing up too quickly, missing out on their chance to be child-like and carefree
- By the time these parents reach out for help, they are often discouraged/hopeless/defensive
- It is preferable to help parents "get back in the driver's seat" without dwelling on theories about "cause"
- Parents may need to vent/feel supported before being able to consider changing their approach
- Often ODD child's negative behaviour and mood comes to dominate the household
- Parents need to "recharge their batteries" in the process of becoming more authoritative in dealing with their child's behaviour

AACAP GUIDELINES FOR ASSESSMENT AND TREATMENT OF ODD

Successful assessment and treatment of ODD require the establishment of therapeutic alliances with the child and the family.

Cultural issues need to be actively considered in diagnosis and treatment.

The assessment of ODD includes information obtained directly from the child and the parents regarding the core symptoms of ODD, age of onset, duration of symptoms, and degree of functional impairment.

Clinician should carefully consider significant comorbid psychiatric conditions when diagnosing and treating ODD.

Clinician may find it helpful to include information obtained independently from multiple outside informants.

The use of specific questionnaires and rating scales may be useful in evaluating children for ODD and tracking their progress.

Clinician should develop an individualized treatment plan based on the specific clinical situation.

Clinician should consider parent intervention based on one of the empirically tested interventions.

Medication may be helpful as adjuncts for symptomatic treatment and to treat comorbid conditions.

Intensive and prolonged treatment may be required if ODD is unusually severe and persistent.

Dramatic, one time, time-limited or short-term interventions are not effective.

PSYCHOSOCIAL MANAGEMENT

Treatment is most effective if it is multimodal, utilized in a variety of settings and includes a home, school, and child component

Parent training program to help manage the child's behaviour

Individual psychotherapy to develop more effective anger management techniques

Family therapy to improve communication between parents and child

Behavioural therapy to reinforce and praise appropriate behaviour and ignore and not reinforce undesired behaviour

PHARMACOLOGICAL INTERVENTION

Medication should not be started until psychological interventions have been attempted

ODD and comorbid ADHD: Stimulants (methylphenidate and dextroamphetamine preparations) and non-stimulants (atomoxetine) may help reduce oppositionality

Atypical antipsychotics may help in aggression

Lithium carbonate reduces aggression and temper outbursts

Carbamazepine may reduce aggressive/explosive behaviour

SSRIs may be helpful for ODD in the context of a mood disorder

NATURAL COURSE OF ODD

The diagnosis of ODD is relatively stable over time, but most children (approximately 67%) will ultimately exit from the diagnosis.

Earlier age of onset of ODD symptoms convey a poor prognosis in terms of progression to CD and ultimately antisocial personality disorder (APD).

Preschool children with ODD are likely to exhibit additional disorders later with increasing age; comorbidity with ADHD, anxiety or mood disorders begin to appear.

PREVENTION OF ODD

For preschool children, home visitation to high-risk families as a preventative intervention has produced positive outcomes.

In school-age children, parent management strategies are the most empirically supported programs.

Social skills, conflict resolution, anger management, cognitive intervention, skills training, vocational training and academic preparation appear to reduce disruptive behaviours.

School-based programs focus on preventing bullying, negative peer pressure, and antisocial behaviour.

CONCLUSION

Oppositional defiant disorder (ODD) is a common clinical problem in children and adolescents. It creates a significant disturbance in social, academic or occupational functioning. ODD is frequently comorbid with other psychiatric conditions and often precedes the development of CD, substance abuse, and severely delinquent behaviour. Treatment of ODD may be particularly problematic and often demands a multimodal approach. There is some evidence that early intervention is preferable, more likely to succeed, and prevents progression into more serious psychopathology.

REFERENCES

American Academy of Child & Adolescent Psychiatry (AACAP). (2009). *Oppositional Defiant Disorder: A Guide for Families.* Retrieved from https://www.aacap.org/App_Themes/AACAP/docs/resource_centers/odd/odd_resource_center_odd_guide.pdf

American Psychiatric Association. (2013). Diagnostic and statistical manual of mental disorders (5th ed.). Arlington, VA, US: American Psychiatric Publishing, Inc.

Canadian ADHD/ADD Resource Alliance (CADDRA). (2010). Canadian ADHD Practice Guidelines (CAP-Guidelines) Third Edition. Retrieved from https://www.caddra.ca/pdfs/caddraGuidelines2011.pdf

Sadock, B. J. (2003). *Kaplan & Sadock's Synopsis of Psychiatry* (9th ed.). B. J. Sadock & V. A. Sadock (Eds.). Philadelphia, Pennsylvania, United States: Lippincott Williams & Wilkins.

Steiner, H. & Remsing, L. (2007). Practice parameter for the assessment and treatment of children and adolescents with oppositional defiant disorder. *J Am Acad Child Adolesc Psychiatry, 46*(1), 126–141.

8. CONDUCT DISORDER

OBJECTIVES

This chapter will discuss the DSM-5 diagnostic criteria for Conduct Disorder (CD). The epidemiology, etiology, assessment, differential diagnosis, comorbidities, critical planning of treatment issues, management, course, protective factors, and prognosis will be highlighted.

INTRODUCTION

Conduct disorder (CD) is a serious diagnosis. The condition is defined as a repetitive and persistent pattern of behaviour that violates the rights of others. CD is manifested in childhood or adolescence and translates to impaired functioning in the classroom, at home, and with peers. Due to their criminal behaviour, CD youth pose a heavy toll on society. Effective treatment and management of conduct disordered youth are crucial.

DSM-5 DIAGNOSTIC CRITERIA FOR CD

Three out of 15 in the past year and one in the past 6 months:
- Bullying
- Animal cruelty
- Destroying other people's property
- Fighting

- Out late at night
- Running away from home
- Actively forcing sex
- Being cruel to people
- Using a weapon
- Setting fires
- Breaking and entering house or car
- Not going to school
- Lying or conning others
- Stealing while confronting a victim
- Stealing without confronting a victim

EPIDEMIOLOGY

The prevalence rate of CD reveals some alarming numbers:

- Isle of Wight community survey: over 3% of 10-yr-olds had CD (Rutter et al., 1970)
- Australia: 6.7% of 10-yr-olds (Connell et al., 1982); New Zealand: 6.9% of 7-yr-olds (McGee et al., 1984)
- Ontario prevalence rate of CD among those 4–16 years old was 5.5% (Offord et al., 1988)

Anywhere between 2% and 16% of school-aged children are believed to meet the diagnostic criteria for CD.

Rates of CD tend to be higher for adolescents (7% for ages 12–16) than for children (4% for ages 4–11).

CD is more prevalent in boys than in girls.

Childhood-onset of CD is considered to be the more serious form of the disorder and generally has a worse prognosis.

ETIOLOGY

CD is complex and multifactorial.

Research has focused on multiple risk factors that contribute to the onset of CD.

These factors are characteristics, events, or processes that increase the likelihood for the onset of the disorder.

RISK FACTORS

Child factors:

- Temperament: child with a more difficult temperament (e.g., negative mood, less adaptability)
- Neuropsychological deficits: deficits in language, memory, motor coordination, and "executive functioning" (e.g., abstract reasoning, planning, attention span and judgment)
- Early behavioural difficulties, early onset of aggression
- Academic difficulties, learning disorders, and lower level of intellectual functioning
- Head injury, seizures, and other neurological insults
- Other psychiatric disorders: ADHD, learning disorders (LD), substance abuse, mood disorders

Parent and family factors:

- Prenatal and perinatal complications: pregnancy and low birth weight, minor birth injury or complication
- Psychopathology and criminal behaviour in the family
- Family history of antisocial personality, alcohol and drug abuse, ADHD, mood disorders, learning disorders

- Poor parenting: coercive parent-child communications, inconsistent discipline, harsh physical punishment, and over-controlling parent
- Poor supervision, few rules
- Impaired quality of family relationships: less warmth, affection, emotional support, and attachment
- Marital discord: conflict or domestic violence
- Large family size: siblings with antisocial behaviour
- Socioeconomic disadvantage: poverty, overcrowding, underemployment, poor housing, financial stress, and lack of supports

School-related factors:

- Inadequate school environment: large classroom with little emphasis on academics
- Poor facilities and workspace
- Infrequent positive feedback from teacher
- Unavailability of teachers and other support staff to deal with student difficulties
- Little emphasis on individual responsibility of students

PROTECTIVE FACTORS

Some children, despite being exposed to high-risk backgrounds, have good psychological outcomes—they are "invulnerable" children

Characteristics of the social group: voluntarily change to a less deviant peer group

Employment may deter antisocial behaviour

Changes of circumstances: improvement of social circumstance

Good relationships: a close, warm, and confiding relationship with one parent/adult

Good experiences: such as school competence or skill development

Coping mechanisms: improving coping through training programs

ESSENTIALS OF ASSESSMENT OF CD

Multi-setting assessments should be made.

Rating scales may be helpful but not diagnostic (e.g., child behavioural checklist).

Ensure a complete psychiatric evaluation for other primary diagnoses or comorbidities.

Perform functional behavioural analysis of the behavioural pattern including baseline and follow up ratings of behaviour.

An educational assessment should be performed if school or learning problems are suspected.

Rule out learning disabilities, cognitive deficits, or sensory loss (hearing or vision problems).

Evaluate the family dynamics, interactions, and communication style, as well as family history of mental health issues.

DIFFERENTIAL DIAGNOSIS

There are no serious diagnostic problems in cases where antisocial behaviour begins at an early age.

Adjustment disorder with disturbance of conduct becomes an important differential diagnosis.

Other differential diagnoses include:
- Substance abuse
- ADHD
- Mood, psychotic, and learning disorders

- Anxiety disorders, such as post-traumatic stress disorder (PTSD)
- Developmental disorders, mental retardation
- Seizure disorders

COMORBIDITY OF CONDUCT DISORDER

"Pure" CD without comorbidities is rare.

The most common comorbidities are ADHD and ODD.

About one-third of ADHD children will have CD and up to 70% of CD children will have ADHD and substance-abuse disorders.

Other common comorbidities include:
- Anxiety disorders
- Bipolar disorder
- Depression
- Adjustment disorder
- Trauma-related disorders
- Developmental disorders

CRITICAL ISSUES IN TREATMENT PLANNING

"Hardcore" CD, where antisocial behaviour first appears before the age of 6 and persists, should be regarded as a lifelong disability requiring lifelong support.

With "hardcore" CD, children do not recover, but with support, patients learn to live with CD without developing major symptomatology. Treatment and support never stop.

Essential factors for treatment to succeed: Presence of family and their willingness to cooperate, to implement behavioural systemic family therapy, are crucial and become an ally to the therapist.

Cognitive and intellectual abilities seem to be a positive factor affecting treatment outcome.

Success of treatment depends on the presence of multiple disabilities (e.g., ADHD, learning disorders) that require well-structured, multi-pronged programming.

MANAGEMENT

Traditional treatments, such as case management, individual psychotherapy, group therapy, and therapeutic community therapy are no more beneficial than no treatment (Romig, 1978).

Treatment is most effective in a variety of settings and includes home, school, and child components.

Early intervention and helping families gain more adaptive methods of relating improve prognosis.

Family ecological-systems approach offers multiple interventions in response to social, cognitive, and interpersonal functioning.

Parent management training: Parents are trained to develop prosocial behaviour in their children's lives; teaching cognitive problem-solving skills. This is a promising psychosocial approach since maladaptive cognitive processes are related to antisocial behaviour.

Anger replacement training: Multimodal psycho-educational intervention for assaultive, hostile adolescents.

Community-based intervention: Aimed at developing prosocial behaviour and better peer relations are a viable alternative to individual treatment.

Helping the offenders to get a job and stay employed.

PROMISING TREATMENT STRATEGIES

Behavioural systemic family therapy: Principles of systemic and behavioural approaches are combined (Gordon et al., 1986).

Cognitive behavioural program (Gordon & Arbuthnot, 1987).

"Think Aloud": a program that relies on modelling and rehearsal of cognitive strategies (Camp & Bush, 1981).

MEDICATION MANAGEMENT OF CD

American Academy of Child and Adolescent Psychiatry (AACAP) indicates that medication alone will be insufficient for managing and treating CD.

Few controlled studies have found that the atypical antipsychotic drug risperidone is effective for reducing aggressive behaviour.

Stimulant and alpha agonist is effective in reducing aggression associated with ADHD and CD.

Mood stabilizers (e.g., lithium and divalproex sodium) have been found to be effective in reducing aggression.

COURSE OF CD

The natural course of conduct disorder has not been carefully studied.

Conduct disorder may stem from very early behavioural patterns: can be described as difficult and irritable infants.

Aggressiveness is the most stable of all early detectable personality characteristics.

Twenty-five-year follow-up of antisocial behaviour found that aggressive behaviour more than any other trait tends to persist once established (Robbins, 1966).

In the youngest group of children, this presents as being argumentative, stubborn, and prone to tantrums, while older children show oppositional behaviour, followed by fire-setting and stealing, and finally truancy, vandalism, and substance abuse.

Which antisocial children are candidates for CD in adolescence and antisocial personality in adulthood?

The critical determining variable is the age at which the CD symptoms first appeared.

Four factors are predictive of chronic delinquency:

1) Frequency of delinquency

2) Age of onset

3) Variety of delinquency

4) Presence of antisocial behaviour in more than one setting

The earlier the age, the greater the likelihood of antisocial behaviour being present in adulthood.

CD may associate in later life with mania, schizophrenia, and obsessive-compulsive disorder.

CD also predicts school dropout, unemployment, financial difficulties, poor interpersonal relationships, and marital conflict.

PROGNOSIS

The best prognosis is for those whose symptoms first appear at 12 years of age or later.

The worst prognosis is for those whose symptoms appear before the age of 6.

Guarded prognosis is for those whose symptoms appear between the ages of 6 and 12 years.

There is a greater success in treating CD when symptoms first appear in adolescence.

Low IQ score and parental antisocial personality disorder predict persistence of CD.

More positive outcomes are predicted by a lower severity of CD, fewer ADHD symptoms, higher verbal IQ, greater family socioeconomic advantage, and biological parents who are not antisocial.

CONCLUSION

Conduct disorder is a serious diagnosis, where the child violates the basic rights of others. No single factor can account for a child's antisocial behaviour. CD is the most difficult disorder to treat in child psychiatry. Conduct disordered youth present the greatest challenge in treatment. Prevention of CD is enhanced by identifying populations at risk and ensuring that children receive the care, attention, and discipline that they need.

REFERENCES

American Psychiatric Association. (2013). Diagnostic and statistical manual of mental disorders (5th ed.). Arlington, VA, US: American Psychiatric Publishing, Inc.

Shamsie, J., Hluchy, C., et al. (1991). Youth with Conduct Disorder: A Challenge to be Met. *The Canadian Journal of Psychiatry, 36*(6), 405–414.

Steiner, H. (1997). Practice Parameters for the Assessment and Treatment of Children and Adolescents With Conduct Disorder. *Journal of the American Academy of Child and Adolescent Psychiatry, 36*(10), 122S–139S.

9. TIC DISORDERS

OBJECTIVES
This chapter outlines the characteristic features and management of tic disorders.

CHARACTERISTIC FEATURES
Brief, rapid, involuntary movements, often resembling fragments of normal behaviour

Worsen with stress, diminish during voluntary activity or mental concentration, and disappear during sleep

Most frequent forms: blinking, sniffing, throat clearing, hitching the shoulder, or throwing the head to the side or backwards

Simple tics (e.g., eye blinking) begin in childhood as nervous mannerisms and disappear spontaneously

TOURETTE'S SYNDROME
Tourette's syndrome is defined as persistent motor and vocal tics that occur simultaneously, lasting over one year.

Multiple motor tics

Vocal tics: sniffing, snorting, involuntary vocalizations, and compulsive utterance of obscenities

May be associated with obsessive-compulsive disorder (OCD) and attention deficit hyperactivity disorder (ADHD)

Often familial clustering

TREATMENT

Simple tics: may respond to benzodiazepines

Tourette's syndrome:
- Noradrenergics
- Clonidine
- Guanfacine
- Dopamine-receptor blockers
- Risperidone
- Haloperidol
- Pimozide

EDUCATION

Patient, family members, teachers

Tourette Syndrome Association

REFERENCES

Jankovic, J. (2001). Tourette's syndrome. *N Engl J Med., 345*(16), 1184–1192.

University of Toronto. (1998). MCCQE Review notes and Lecture series. Toronto, Canada: Faculty of Medicine, University of Toronto.

10. FETAL ALCOHOL SYNDROME

OBJECTIVES

This chapter will discuss the characteristic features of fetal alcohol syndrome (FAS). Confirmed maternal exposure to alcohol, atypical presentation, diagnosis, and maternal screening of alcohol use/abuse will be discussed. Secondary and tertiary prevention of maternal alcohol abuse and treatment for children with FAS will also be described.

INTRODUCTION

Fetal alcohol syndrome (FAS) is a common and fully preventable disabling condition that can affect children from all social classes.

Alcohol is a teratogen and there is no conclusive evidence regarding a safe level of alcohol use during pregnancy.

The severity of the disability is proportionate to alcohol exposure.

Obtaining accurate information about alcohol consumption can be difficult and requires appropriate direct questioning.

With proper inquiry and appropriate counselling, physicians can help most pregnant women stop or reduce alcohol consumption.

FAS WITH CONFIRMED MATERNAL ALCOHOL EXPOSURE

Confirmed maternal alcohol exposure: substantial regular or episodic intake

Characteristic pattern of facial anomalies, e.g., short palpebral fissure, thin upper lip, smooth philtrum, recessed or flat midface

Growth retardation in either prenatal or postnatal period or low birth weight to height in infancy and early childhood

Central nervous system (CNS) and neurodevelopmental abnormalities:

- Decreased cranial size at birth, structural brain abnormalities, e.g., microcephaly, partial or complete agencies of the corpus callosum, neural migration defects

- Hard or soft neurological signs, e.g., poor fine-motor skills, poor hand-eye coordination, poor tendon gate, hearing loss

FAS without confirmed maternal exposure includes a characteristic pattern of facial anomalies, growth retardation, neurodevelopmental abnormalities, hard and soft neurological signs.

PARTIAL OR ATYPICAL FAS WITH CONFIRMED MATERNAL ALCOHOL EXPOSURE

Some facial anomaly, growth retardation, neurodevelopmental anomalies.

Evidence of a complex pattern of behaviour or cognitive abnormalities inconsistent with developmental level and cannot be explained by familial background or environment alone, e.g., learning difficulties, poor school performance, poor impulse control.

Poor social perception, deficit in language, poor capacity for abstraction, special deficit in math skills, problems in memory, attention or judgment.

SCREENING FOR ALCOHOL USE/ABUSE

Do you use alcohol? If the answer is No: low risk

If the answer is Yes: at-risk patient. Apply secondary prevention strategies (see below).

Brief interventions:

    a) Advise by providing personalized feedback to the patient.

    b) Advise the patient to stop or reduce drinking.

    c) Assist by providing the patient with material to facilitate the change.

    d) Refer to appropriate resources.

Standard screening test for alcohol use:

- T-ACE questionnaire
- Tolerance: How many drinks does it take to make you feel high?
    - Score 2 for more than two drinks
    - Score 0 for two or fewer drinks
- Annoyance: Have people annoyed you by criticizing your drinking?
    - Score 1 if yes
- Cut down: Have you felt you ought to cut down on your drinking?
    - Score 1 if yes

- Eye-opener: Have you ever had a drink first thing in the morning to steady your nerves or get rid of a hangover?
  ○ Score 1 if yes
- High-risk score = 2 or more points

High-risk patient:

a) Urgent referral to specialized resources (priority given to prenatal patients)
b) Continued follow-up and support

(Modified from the Institute of Medicine (US) Division of Behavioural Science & Mental Disorder Committee to Study FAS, 1996)

PREVENTION OF FAS

Primary prevention strategies:

- Community education and individual support with complete avoidance of alcohol prior to conception
- Ask all female patients of child-bearing age the basic question about their use of alcohol
- Promote zero tolerance for alcohol when planning or during pregnancy
- Discuss avoidance of conception if alcohol is being consumed. Refer women (or couple) for alcohol counselling and treatment if they have had an FAS child
- Be aware of and use promotional materials in offices and as handouts for patients
- Be aware of access to community resources

Secondary prevention strategies:
- Screening for identification of the persons at risk; intervention program services for pregnant women who may be at risk for having a child with FAS
- Counsel pregnant women who are using alcohol about the effect on their fetus and their own health
- Counsel pregnant women regarding the benefits of stopping or at least significantly reducing the use of alcohol at any time during pregnancy
- Refer pregnant women for appropriate treatment who are using alcohol

Tertiary prevention strategies:
- Aimed at reducing the complications, impairment, and disabilities caused by FAS
- Proper diagnosis facilitates treatment and services for children with FAS
- Diagnosis also facilitates primary and secondary prevention for subsequent pregnancies

COMORBIDITY

Comorbid conditions commonly include:
- Learning disabilities
- Attention deficit hyperactivity disorder
- Conduct disorder
- Secondary disabilities

TREATMENT FOR FAS CHILDREN

Individualized and multidisciplinary approach including:
- Diagnostic assessment
- Social services
- Educational support
- Rehabilitation

CONCLUSION

There is no safe amount of alcohol consumption during pregnancy. Counselling women and couples planning or during pregnancy about the effects of alcohol use are imperative to encourage the reduction or complete cessation of alcohol consumption. Individualized and multidisciplinary care is required to treat children with FAS.

REFERENCES

Alberta Partnership on Fetal Alcohol Syndrome. (2000). Prevention & Diagnosis of Fetal Alcohol Syndrome. Retrieved from http://www.dronet.org/lineeguida/ligu_pdf/feto_al2.pdf

Institute of Medicine. (1996). Fetal Alcohol Syndrome: Diagnosis, Epidemiology, Prevention, and Treatment. Institute of Medicine, National Academy Press, Washington, D.C., U.S.A. Retrieved from http://www.come-over.to/FAS/IOMsummary.htm

11. COMMON ANXIETY DISORDERS IN CHILDHOOD AND ADOLESCENCE

OBJECTIVES

This chapter will discuss the essential concepts related to separation anxiety, selective mutism, panic disorder, agoraphobia, generalized anxiety disorder, specific phobias, social anxiety, and post-traumatic stress disorder. The epidemiology of various anxiety disorders, characteristic features, diagnosis, and management will also be highlighted.

INTRODUCTION

Most children experience various fears throughout their childhood. Some of the fears are specific to the developmental stage the child is in.

In contrast to fear, anxiety is defined as an anticipatory response to a perceived threat, either internal or external.

Both fear and anxiety are characterized by the distressing "fight-or-flight" reaction and other physiological responses that may affect multiple systems, such as cardiac, gastrointestinal, and neurological systems.

SEPARATION ANXIETY DISORDER (SAD)

Common anxiety disorder of children, characterized by extreme anxiety and worry concerning separation from home or primary caregivers

Often diagnosed in preschool or kindergarten when a child experiences separation from an attachment figure

Generally, a disorder of childhood and remits with advancing age but may occur in adults as well

Essential Concepts of SAD

Usually presents with somatic complaints, e.g., headache or stomachache to avoid leaving home

About three-quarters of children with SAD exhibit school avoidance

Children with SAD experience unrealistic fears that they or their parents will be injured, kidnapped, or killed

Children with SAD are disabled by their inability to sleep alone, attend school, or stay at camp

Epidemiology

Affects 2.4% to 4.7% of the population of children

Male to female ratio almost equal

Anxiety disorders tend to run in families

Etiology

Likely precipitated by the interaction of genetic, temperament, family dynamics, and other environmental factors

Assessment

Assessment includes a standard complete psychiatric evaluation. Multiple informants are crucial.

A parent may need to be present for the entire interview of the child if he or she is unable to separate.

Assessment should focus on symptoms of anxiety and/or mood disorders in both the child and parents.

Differential diagnosis includes other anxiety disorders, depressive disorders, and pervasive developmental disorders or psychosis.

Diagnosis

Three out of the following eight symptoms are required:

1. Physical symptoms and complaints with anticipated separation
2. Event anxiety
3. Sleep difficulties
4. Concerned with harm to attachment figures
5. Nightmares
6. Afraid of being alone
7. Going to school or out of home difficult
8. Separation fears

The fear, anxiety, or avoidance is persistent, lasting at least 4 weeks in children and adolescents and typically 6 months or more in adults. This causes clinically significant impairment.

Management of SAD

Treatment is multimodal and includes parents, school intervention, and medication if symptoms are severe and disabling.

Parent must be involved in therapy to reassure the child as he or she achieves more independence and autonomy.

Psychosocial intervention includes cognitive behavioural and psychodynamic psychotherapy, combined with parent guidance, behavioural modification, and family therapy.

Psychotherapy combined with parent guidance and school consultation is more effective.

Child benefits from learning relaxation skills and sleep hygiene.

Medication treatment is typically selective serotonin reuptake inhibitors (SSRI). Benzodiazepines may be indicated for school refusal due to high anxiety.

SELECTIVE MUTISM

Now included in DSM-5 as an anxiety disorder

Epidemiology

Prevalence is less than 1% for school-age children

Girls are thought to be affected twice as often as boys

Onset in preschool years, although it is not identified until starting school

The child with selective mutism consistently does not speak in specific social situations in which there is an expectation for speaking, such as school

Child speaks well in familiar environments, e.g., at home with family members

Symptoms must persist for at least one month and be severe enough to negatively impact educational and interpersonal functioning

Treatment

Behavioural therapy

Parental counselling: Parents and siblings are discouraged from routinely talking for the child

SSRI

PANIC DISORDER

Epidemiology

Incidence of panic disorder in children and adolescents is between 0.5% and 5%

Onset is most often in late adolescence

More common in girls than boys

Diagnosis

Recurrent unexpected panic attacks followed by at least one month of persistent concern about another panic attack, about consequences, or significant behavioural changes related to attack

Panic attack—a discrete period of intense fear in which four of the following symptoms develop abruptly and reach a peak within minutes:

- Palpitations
- Sweating
- Trembling or shaking
- Shortness of breath or smothering sensation
- Choking feeling
- Chest pain/discomfort
- Nausea or abdominal distress

- Feeling dizzy, unsteady, lightheaded or faint
- Derealization or depersonalization
- Fear of losing control or going crazy
- Fear of dying
- Paresthesias (tingling, pins-and-needles sensation)
- Chills or hot flashes

Symptoms are unexpected with no obvious precipitant

Rule out other causes: drugs (amphetamine, caffeine, alcohol) or medical condition (hyperthyroidism, mitral valve prolapse, hypoglycemia, pheochromocytoma)

Clinical course: chronic but episodic

Complication: depression

Treatment

Physical exam and review of systems; medical workup as indicated

Supportive psychotherapy, cognitive-behavioural therapy (CBT)

Minor tranquillizer, SSRI antidepressant

Prognosis

Six to ten years post-treatment: 30% well, 40%–50% improved, 20%–30% no change or worse

AGORAPHOBIA

Separate diagnosis from panic disorder in DSM-5

Anxiety about being in places or situations from which escape might be difficult (or embarrassing) or where help may not be available in the event of having an unexpected panic attack

Fears commonly involve clusters of situations like being out alone, being in a crowd, standing in a line, travelling on a bus

Situations are avoided, endured with anxiety or panic, or require a companion

Treatment: As per panic disorder + behavioural therapy

GENERALIZED ANXIETY DISORDER (GAD)

Epidemiology
Three to six percent of youth

Diagnosis
Excessive anxiety and worry for at least 6 months about a number of events and activities

Difficult to control the worry

Three or more of the following six symptoms:
- Restlessness, feeling keyed up, or on edge
- Easy fatigability
- Difficulty concentrating
- Irritability
- Muscle tension
- Sleep disturbance

Treatment
Cognitive behavioural therapy (CBT)
Relaxation therapy
SSRI, NSRI, buspirone

Prognosis

Chronically anxious child/youth becomes less so with age

Depends on premorbid personality functioning, stability in relations, study, and severity of environmental stress

SPECIFIC PHOBIA

Epidemiology

Estimated at around 5% in children and adolescents

Phobias are more common in girls

Onset is common in childhood

Features

Marked and persistent fear of clearly discernible circumscribed objects or situations

Exposure to stimulus provokes immediate anxiety response

Diagnosis

Only made if phobia interferes with daily routine, functioning, or causes marked distress

Types

Animal

Natural environment (heights, storms)

Blood, injection

Situational

Other (loud noises, clowns)

Treatment

Cognitive behavioural therapy (systematic desensitization, flooding)

SSRI Antidepressant

SOCIAL ANXIETY DISORDER

Epidemiology

Affects 1% to 2% of children and adolescents

Social anxiety disorder occurs in childhood and adolescence

More common in girls than in boys

Symptoms

Marked and persistent fear of social performance in situations in which embarrassment may occur, e.g., public speaking, public washroom use, blushing in public

Anxiety persists or increases (as opposed to normal performance anxiety which decreases)

Symptoms must persist for 6 months

Treatment

Anxiety-reducing strategy

Cognitive behavioural therapy (CBT)

Social-skills training

SSRI antidepressant

Beta-blocker for performance anxiety

Prognosis

Chronic

POST-TRAUMATIC STRESS DISORDER (PTSD)

Described in trauma and stressor-related disorder groups in DSM-5.

Epidemiology

30% to 60% of children develop PTSD following a disaster

25% to 30% of children develop PTSD after a road traffic accident. Significant number after any abuse.

Lifetime prevalence of PTSD is 8%

Diagnosis

An event experienced involving threat of death/serious injury or threat to physical integrity of self or other

Response involves intense fear, helplessness or horror

Traumatic event is persistently re-experienced through one or more of the following:

- Recurrent, distressing recollections (images, thoughts)
- Recurrent distressing dreams
- Acting or feeling as if the event is happening again (flashback)
- Distress at exposure to cues that resemble the event
- Persistent avoidance of stimuli associated with trauma and numbing of general responsiveness
- Persistent symptoms of increased arousal (insomnia, irritability, difficulty concentrating, hyper-vigilance, exaggerated startle response)

Symptoms present for greater than one month

For children under 6 years of age, separate diagnostic criteria have been described in DSM-5

Treatment

Cognitive behavioural therapy (systematic desensitization, relaxation techniques, thought stopping)

SSRI antidepressant

Beta blocker for autonomic symptoms

CONCLUSION

Most children experience various fears and often anxiety. However, anxiety disorders may have a significant psychosocial impact on a child or adolescent. Identification of anxieties and their management improve functioning at school, interaction with peers, and dynamics at home.

REFERENCES

American Psychiatric Association. (2013). Diagnostic and statistical manual of mental disorders (5th ed.). Arlington, VA, US: American Psychiatric Publishing, Inc.

Coghill, D., Graham, J., & Bonnar, S., et al. (2009). *Child and Adolescent Psychiatry*. Oxford, United Kingdom: Oxford University Press.

Stubbe, D. (2007). *Child and Adolescent Psychiatry*. Philadelphia, Pennsylvania, United States: Lippincott Williams & Wilkins.

University of Toronto. (1998). MCCQE Review notes and Lecture series. Toronto, Canada: Faculty of Medicine, University of Toronto.

12. CHILDHOOD AND ADOLESCENT DEPRESSION

OBJECTIVES

This chapter will discuss the epidemiology, etiology, clinical manifestations, and DSM-5 diagnostic criteria for childhood and adolescent depression. Subtypes of depression and risk factors will be highlighted. Assessment, differential diagnosis, and comorbidity will be described. Controversy surrounding the use of antidepressants, including side effects in children and adolescents will be discussed. Principles of the treatment of depression, as well as depression and suicidality, the course of depression, prognosis, and prevention, will also be discussed.

INTRODUCTION

Understanding and treating childhood and adolescent depression is a complex and challenging dilemma for families, clinicians and teens themselves. Depressive disorders are often familial and recurrent illnesses associated with a high prevalence and an increased psychosocial morbidity and mortality. There have been significant developments in the understanding of depression in children and adolescents over the past few years, including an increased recognition that depressive illness occurs in this age group. This has also led to the emergence of newer antidepressants, leading to the controversy of their use in children and adolescents.

EPIDEMIOLOGY OF DEPRESSION

Over the past six decades, the prevalence of depression has increased and the age at the time of diagnosis has decreased. The prevalence of depression is estimated to be approximately 2% in children and 4% to 8% in adolescents with a male to female ratio of 1:1 during childhood and 1:2 during adolescence. Approximately 5% to 10% of children and adolescents have subsyndromal symptoms of depression. These youth have considerable psychosocial impairment, high family loading for depression, and an increased risk of suicide and depression. A few epidemiological studies on dysthymic disorder (DD) have reported a prevalence of 0.6% to 1.7% in children and 1.6% to 8% in adolescents.

ETIOLOGY OF DEPRESSION

High-risk adoption and twin studies have shown that depression is a familial disorder, which is caused by the interaction of genetic and environmental factors.

Genetic factors may influence the functioning of the hypothalamic-pituitary-adrenal axis and functioning of the serotonin, cholinergic, and noradrenergic systems, which show deregulation under stress in depression.

The onset and recurrences of depression may be moderated or mediated by the presence of stressors such as losses, abuse, neglect, and ongoing conflict and frustrations.

Anxiety, substance abuse, ADHD, eating disorders, medical illness (e.g., diabetes), use of medications, biological, and sociocultural factors have also been related to the development and maintenance of depressive symptomatology.

CLINICAL PRESENTATION

The overall clinical picture of depression in children and adolescents is similar to the clinical picture in adults, but there are some differences that could be attributed to the child's physical, emotional, cognitive and social developmental stages:

- Children may have mood lability, irritability, low frustration tolerance, temper tantrums, somatic complaints, and/or social withdrawal instead of verbalizing feelings of depression.
- Children also tend to have fewer melancholic symptoms, delusions, and suicide attempts than depressed adults.

DSM-5 DIAGNOSTIC CRITERIA FOR DEPRESSION

To be diagnosed with clinical depression, a child or adolescent must have at least two weeks of persistent change in mood manifested by either depressed or irritable mood and/or loss of interest or pleasure plus a group of symptoms including wishing to be dead, suicidal ideation or attempts, increased or decreased appetite, weight or sleep, and decreased activity, concentration, energy or self-worth or exaggerated guilt.

These symptoms must represent a change from previous functioning and produce impairment in relationships or performance of activities.

Furthermore, symptoms must not be attributable only to substance abuse, use of medications, other psychiatric illness, or medical illness.

SUBTYPES OF DEPRESSION

There are various subtypes of depression that may have treatment and prognostic implications. Psychotic depression has been associated with a family history of bipolar and psychotic depression, more severe depression, greater long-term morbidity, resistance to antidepressant monotherapy, and most notably, increased risk of bipolar disorder.

Depression can be manifested with atypical symptoms such as increased reactivity to rejection, lethargy, increased appetite, craving for carbohydrates, and hypersomnia. Patients with seasonal affective disorder mainly have symptoms of depression during the season with less daylight.

PERSISTENT DEPRESSIVE DISORDER "DYSTHYMIA"

Persistent depressive disorder consists of a persistent long-term change of mood that generally is less intense but more chronic than in a major depressive episode (MDE). This disorder is often overlooked and misdiagnosed, but it causes as much or more psychosocial impairment.

For DSM-5 diagnosis of persistent depressive disorder, a child must have a depressed mood or irritability on most days for a period of one year and symptoms including at least two of the following: change of appetite or weight, changes in sleep, problems with decision making or concentration, and low self-esteem, energy, and hope.

RISK FACTORS FOR DEPRESSION

Individual factors:
- Low self-esteem
- Lack of emotional support
- Poor social or interpersonal skills
- Conflicting peer relationships
- Bullying

- Identity problems
- Confusion related to sexual orientation
- Female gender
- Poor body image
- Lack of academic performance
- Antisocial behaviour, particularly aggressive impulsive behaviour
- Alcohol and substance abuse
- Early adversity
- Poor care and/or neglect
- Physical, emotional, and sexual abuse

Parental separation, divorce, or family conflict

Family factors:
- Inadequate or excessive parental authority
- High or low family expectations
- Parental mental health problems and alcohol and substance misuse
- Socioeconomic factors

Deliberate self-harm is reported to occur equally across all socioeconomic groups in adolescence. This is in contrast to the adult population where higher rates occur in lower socioeconomic groups.

ASSESSMENT OF DEPRESSION

Assessment of children and adolescents should routinely include screening questions about depressive symptomatology.

While screening instruments can be very useful, it is important to know that none of these questionnaires are designed to diagnose depression.

The most widely used and best validated self-report instruments for assessing depressive symptoms in children are the Children's Depression Inventory (CDI), Beck Depression Inventory for Youth (BDIY), and the Mood and Feelings Questionnaire (MFQ).

If screening indicates significant depressive symptomatology, the clinician should perform a thorough evaluation to determine the presence of depression and other comorbid psychiatric and medical disorders.

Evaluation must include the assessment for the presence of harm to self or others. It is also vital for clinicians to evaluate for any prior history of suicidal behaviours and to evaluate this frequently in subsequent visits.

The evaluation should assess for the presence of ongoing or past exposure to negative events, the environment in which depression is developing, support, and family psychiatric history.

Once a diagnosis is made, patients and families need to be educated about the illness and the options available for treatment.

If medication is required, families and patients need to be fully informed about the risks and benefits of antidepressant treatment.

Clinician should maintain a confidential relationship with the child or adolescent while developing collaborative relationships with parents, medical providers, other mental health professionals, and appropriate school personnel.

DIFFERENTIAL DIAGNOSIS OF DEPRESSION

Psychiatric conditions

Adjustment disorder

Depressive phase of emerging bipolar disorder

Bereavement

Persistent depressive disorder

Substance abuse

Anxiety disorder

Attention deficit hyperactivity disorder

Oppositional defiant disorder

Pervasive developmental disorder

MEDICAL DISORDERS

Hypothyroidism

Anemia

Certain cancers

Autoimmune diseases

Premenstrual dysphoric disorders

Chronic fatigue syndrome

Infectious etiologies: HIV, hepatitis, mononucleosis

Medications: corticosteroids, beta blockers, contraceptives, etc.

COMORBIDITY OF DEPRESSION

Both depression and dysthymia are usually accompanied by other psychiatric and medical conditions.

Forty percent to ninety percent of youth with depressive disorder also have other psychiatric disorders.

Most common comorbid diagnoses are anxiety disorders, followed by disruptive disorders and substance use disorders.

Depression and dysthymia usually manifest after the onset of other psychiatric disorders, e.g., anxiety.

Depression increases the risk of the development of non-mood psychiatric disorders, e.g., conduct and substance-abuse disorders.

CONTROVERSY ABOUT THE USE OF ANTIDEPRESSANTS IN CHILDREN AND ADOLESCENTS

There has been much recent controversy about the use of SSRIs and other antidepressants in children and adolescents.

The data suggests that antidepressants pose a 4% risk versus a 2% risk in placebo of suicidal thinking or behaviour.

This prompted the FDA to issue a "Black Box" warning for suicidality for all antidepressants.

Notably, there were no completed suicides in the study samples.

We do not entirely understand the finding of "suicidality" as a noted side effect of SSRIs.

CLINICAL RECOMMENDATIONS FOR USE OF ANTIDEPRESSANTS

Family and patient need to be fully informed about the possible risk of the emergence of suicidal behaviours with antidepressant treatment.

Antidepressants should be initiated at a low dose (e.g., equivalent of 5 mg to 10 mg of fluoxetine) with increases every 2 weeks if no significant adverse events emerge.

Patient should be closely monitored for worsening depression, worsening or new onset of suicidality and other side effects.

The FDA suggests weekly face-to-face monitoring for the first 4 weeks of antidepressant treatment or with any subsequent dose adjustments in children and adolescents.

MEDICATION TREATMENT FOR DEPRESSION

Fluoxetine, an SSRI, is the best-studied of all antidepressants. It is the only one to show a significant advantage over placebo in terms of efficacy for depression in children and adolescents.

Citalopram, escitalopram, and sertraline have some positive studies as well.

Randomized controlled trials (RCTs) have shown no difference between venlafaxine or mirtazapine and placebo.

Open-level studies have suggested bupropion's effectiveness in treating adolescent depression with or without ADHD.

RCTs, as well as meta-analyses, have shown that tricyclic antidepressants are no more efficacious than a placebo for the treatment of child and adolescent depression and should not be used as a first-line medication.

SIDE EFFECTS OF ANTIDEPRESSANTS

Overall, SSRIs and other novel antidepressants are well tolerated by children and adolescents with few short-term side effects.

The common side effects include gastrointestinal symptoms, sleep changes (e.g., insomnia or somnolence, vivid dreams, nightmares, and impaired sleep), restlessness, akathisia diaphoresis, headaches, increase or decrease in appetite, and sexual dysfunction.

Approximately 3% to 8% of children may show increased impulsivity, agitation, irritability, silliness, and "behavioural activation."

More rarely, the use of antidepressants has been associated with serotonin syndrome, easy bruising, and epistaxis.

Venlafaxine may cause elevated blood pressure, mirtazapine may increase appetite and weight, trazodone may cause priapism, and Wellbutrin may cause seizures.

PRINCIPLES OF TREATMENT FOR DEPRESSION

Treatment of depressive disorders should always include an acute and continuation phase. Some children may also require maintenance treatment.

Each phase of treatment should include psychoeducation, supportive management, family and school involvement.

Education, support, and case management appear to be sufficient treatment for the management of depressed children and adolescents with an uncomplicated or brief depression or with mild psychosocial impairment.

Children and adolescents who do not respond to supportive psychotherapy or who have more complicated depression may need a more specific type of psychotherapy and/or antidepressants. To consolidate the response to the acute treatment and avoid relapses, treatment should always be continued for 6 to 12 months.

Depressed patients with psychosis, seasonal depression, and bipolar disorder may require more specific treatments.

Treatment of depressive disorder should include the management of comorbid conditions.

During all treatment phases, clinicians should arrange frequent follow-up contact that allows sufficient time to monitor the subject's clinical status, environmental conditions, and if appropriate, medication side effects.

For a child or adolescent who is not responding to appropriate pharmacological and/or psychotherapeutic treatments, the clinician may need to consider factors associated with poor response.

Parent and child psychoeducation: about depression as a disease, treatment, what the patient and family can do to decrease depression, education around safety, and need to secure medications. Always ask about guns. Be sure there are none or they are locked.

Hospitalization: if the child is suicidal or engaging in self-destructive behaviours, hospitalization needs to be considered.

DEPRESSION AND SUICIDALITY

Studies have found that 85% of depressed youth report significant suicidal ideation and 32% report a history of one or more suicidal attempts.

The rates for suicide increase markedly from children aged 5–14 years (0.61 per 100,000) to teens aged 15–19 years (7.26 per 100,000).

For teens aged 15–19 years, boys had higher suicide rates than girls, whereas girls had higher rates of unsuccessful attempts.

Of the adolescents who completed suicide, 35% to 45% had a previous suicidal attempt. Longitudinal follow-up study of clinically depressed adolescents found a completed suicide rate of almost 8%.

Several factors have been identified as increasing the risk of suicidal behaviour and completion. Frequent suicidal thoughts and previous suicidal behaviour are the strongest predictors for suicide attempts and behaviours. The more severe the suicidal thoughts, the greater the likelihood of an attempt within the next year.

The risk of suicidal behaviour increases if there is a history of suicide attempts, comorbid psychiatric disorders, impulsivity, aggression, availability of lethal agents, exposure to negative events (e.g., physical and sexual abuse), violence, and a family history of suicide.

COURSE OF DEPRESSION

Untreated depressive episode for clinic-referred youth typically lasts for 7 to 9 months. In community samples, it is about 1 to 2 months.

Approximately 90% of cases of depression remit within 1 to 2 years from onset. However, 6% to 10% of episodes become more persistent.

A large North American study found that 12% of adolescents with depression relapsed within 1 year and 33% relapsed within 4 years.

Relapse of depression occurs in 20% to 60% of adolescents within 2 years and up to 70% of adolescents within 5 years.

Dysthymia lasts on average 3 to 4 years and patients have an increased risk of developing depression and substance-abuse disorders.

Between 40% and 70% of depressed adolescents will experience a recurrence of depression in adulthood.

After an acute episode of depression, a slow and gradual improvement of psychosocial functioning may occur unless there is a relapse or recurrence.

Psychosocial difficulties frequently persist after the remission of a depressive episode.

Children and adolescents with depressive disorders are at high risk of substance abuse, legal problems, exposure to negative life events, physical illness, early pregnancy and poor academic functioning.

Comorbid psychopathology, poor family functioning, parental psychopathology, and low socioeconomic status may affect the psychosocial functioning of depressed youths.

PROGNOSIS OF DEPRESSION

If untreated, depression may affect the development of a child's emotional, cognitive, and social skills, and interfere with family relationships.

Suicide attempts and completion are among the most significant and devastating sequelae of depression.

Maintaining factors that predict a longer duration of an episode include greater severity of initial depression, presence of ongoing chronic adversity, comorbid psychiatric disorders, psychiatric illness in parents, and poor psychosocial functioning.

PREVENTION OF DEPRESSION

Prevention of the onset or recurrence of depression should include the amelioration of risk factors.

Children with risk factors for depression should have access to early service interventions.

Programs that include populations at risk are more effective than those targeting general populations.

Anxiety disorder is a precursor of depression. Treatment of anxiety may reduce the onset and recurrence of depression.

Early-onset dysthymia is associated with an increased risk of depression, indicating the need for early treatment.

Lifestyle modifications include regular and adequate sleep, exercise, a coping plan for stress, the pursuit of enjoyable and meaningful activities, and avoidance of stressful situations.

It is important to educate caregivers, school personnel, pediatricians, and youth about the warning signs of depressive disorders and appropriate sources of assessment and treatment.

Early identification and vigorous treatment of mothers with depression are associated with significantly fewer new psychiatric diagnoses and higher remission rates of existing disorders in children.

CONCLUSION

Depression in children and adolescents is a relatively common, multifactorial, recurrent illness. Evidence-based research supports the effectiveness of psychotherapeutic intervention and medication management. Early identification and effective treatment may reduce the impact of depression on the family, social, and academic functioning in children and youth and may reduce the risk of suicide, substance abuse, and persistence of depressive disorders in adulthood.

REFERENCES

American Psychiatric Association. (2013). Diagnostic and statistical manual of mental disorders (5th ed.). Arlington, VA, US: American Psychiatric Publishing, Inc.

Birhamer, B. & David, B. (2007). Practice parameter for the assessment and treatment of children and adolescents with depressive disorders. *Journal of the American Academy of Child and Adolescent Psychiatry, 46*(11), 1503–1526.

Carr, A. (2008). Depression in young people: description, assessment and evidence-based treatment. *Dev Neurorehabil, 11*(1), 3–15.

Jackson, B. & Lurie, S. (2006). Adolescent depression: challenges and opportunities: a review and current recommendations for clinical practice. *Adv Pediatr., 53*, 111–163.

Richardson, L. P. & Katzenellenbogen, R. (2005). Childhood and adolescent depression: the role of primary care providers in diagnosis and treatment. *Curr Probl Pediatr Adolesc Health Care, 35*(1), 6–24.

Stubbe, D. (2007). *Child and Adolescent Psychiatry.* Philadelphia, Pennsylvania, United States: Lippincott Williams & Wilkins.

13. PEDIATRIC BIPOLAR MOOD DISORDER

OBJECTIVES

This chapter will discuss the DSM-5 diagnostic criteria for bipolar mood disorder. Disruptive mood dysregulation disorder, a new addition to DSM-5 will be described. Difficulties in diagnosing children with bipolar disorder will be explained, including risk factors. Features unique to youth with bipolar illness will be discussed. Assessment, management, and treatment of bipolar disorder will be described. Lastly, outcomes of pediatric bipolar disorder and a treatment strategy to move beyond episodes will be discussed.

INTRODUCTION

Bipolar disorder is a devastating mood disorder that may require lifelong treatment. Symptoms of bipolar disorder usually arise during adolescence. In many cases, as long as 5 to 10 years may elapse before the formal diagnosis is made. Management of this disorder is complicated by a number of factors, including high proportions of bipolar patients with comorbid conditions and non-compliance.

DSM-5 DIAGNOSTIC CRITERIA OF DISRUPTIVE MOOD DISREGULATION DISORDER

Children with chronic, severe irritability (explosive outbursts) have been given a diagnosis of "disruptive mood dysregulation disorder" (formerly temper dysregulation disorder diagnosis).

A) Very severe, recurrent temper outbursts manifested verbally (rages) and/or behaviourally (physical aggression)

B) Temper outbursts are inconsistent with developmental level

C) Temper outbursts occur 3 or more times per week

D) The mood between temper outbursts is persistently irritable or angry

E) Criteria A–D have been present for 12 or more months and have not lasted 3 or more months without all symptoms in criteria A–D

F) Criteria A–D are present in at least two or more settings

G) The diagnosis should not be made for the first time before age 6 and after age 18 years

H) By history and observation, the age of onset of criteria A–E is before 10 years of age

I) Manic or hypomanic symptoms have not been met

J) The behaviours do not occur exclusively during an episode of major depressive disorder and are not better explained by another mental disorder

K) Symptoms are not attributable to another medical condition or effects of substance abuse

TREATMENT APPROACH FOR DISRUPTIVE MOOD DYSREGULATION DISORDER

Good diagnostic assessment

It matters if ADHD, anxiety, ASD, learning disability, or something else is underlying the rage

Maximize the treatment of the base condition

If symptoms remain, add another medication (e.g., atypical antipsychotics or mood stabilizer)

Keep careful records of frequency, intensity, number, and duration of episodes

MANIA: DSM-5 CRITERIA

A) Distinct period of abnormally elevated, expansive or irritable mood and persistently increased goal-directed activity or high energy lasting at least one week (or any duration if hospitalization is necessary)

B) During episode, three or more of the following symptoms have been present to a significant degree:

1) Inflated self-esteem or grandiosity
2) Decreased need for sleep
3) Pressure in speech
4) Flight of ideas
5) Distractibility
6) Psychomotor agitation
7) Excessive involvement in a pleasurable activity that has a high potential for painful consequences

C) Mood disturbance is severe enough to cause sufficient impairment in functioning

D) The episode is not attributable to another medical condition, drug abuse, or medication

HYPOMANIA DSM-5 CRITERIA

A) Distinct period of persistently elevated, expansive or irritable mood lasting at least 4 consecutive days and present most days

B) During mood disturbance three or more of seven manic symptoms from mania episode (see section B above) are present

C) The episode is associated with a change in functioning level

D) Disturbance of mood and functioning is observable by others

E) Episode is not severe enough to cause marked impairment in functioning to necessitate hospitalization and there are no psychotic features

F) The episode is not attributable to drug abuse or medication

MAJOR DEPRESSIVE EPISODE DSM-5 CRITERIA

A) Five or more of the following symptoms are present in the same 2-week period with at least one symptom of either (1) depressed mood or (2) loss of interest or pleasure:

1) Depressed mood, or
2) Loss of interest or pleasure, and
3) Weight loss or gain
4) Insomnia or hypersomnia
5) Psychomotor agitation or retardation
6) Fatigue or loss of energy

7) Worthlessness or guilty feeling

8) Poor concentration or indecisiveness

9) Suicidal ideation, plan, or attempt

B) Symptoms cause significant impairment in functioning in social, occupational, or other areas in life

C) The episode is not due to use of a substance/or another medical condition

Criteria A–C above constitute a major depressive episode (MDE). Symptoms are not due to bereavement.

CYCLOTHYMIC DISORDER

A) For at least 2 years (1 year for children and adolescents) numerous periods of hypomanic and depressive symptoms that do not meet criteria for hypomanic or major depressive episode

B) During the above periods, hypomanic and depressive symptoms have been present for at least half the time and individual has not been symptom-free for more than 2 months at a time

C) Criteria for major depressive, manic or hypomanic episode has never been met

D) Symptoms in criteria A are not better explained by schizophrenia spectrum disorders or depressive illness

The episode is not attributable to drug abuse or medication. Symptoms cause significant functioning impairment.

EPIDEMIOLOGY

Twenty percent onset in adolescence: peak incidence is 15–19 years old

Prepuberty 0.2% to 0.4%; Adolescent incidence 1%

Equal sex distribution

Twenty to thirty percent of depressed adolescents switch to mania

Eighty to ninety percent have a recurrence after the first episode

Sixth leading cause of disability

At least 25% attempt and 15% complete suicide

WHY IS BIPOLAR DISORDER DIFFICULT TO DIAGNOSE IN CHILDREN AND YOUTH?

Developmental variation in adolescent mood disorder and in their presenting symptoms

DSM-V time constraint; adult criteria not particularly helpful with children

Symptoms overlap with other diagnoses, e.g., ADHD

Identifying episode's onset and offset is very difficult

High prevalence of mixed and dysphoric states, less classic euphoric mania, more mood lability and irritability

RISK FACTORS THAT MAY PREDICT EVENTUAL MANIC EPISODE

Depressive episode with rapid onset of psychomotor retardation and psychotic features

Family history of affective disorder, especially bipolar disorder (genetic loading)

History of mania/hypomania after treatment with antidepressants

PARENT-REPORTED SYMPTOMS IN CHILDREN WHO MAY ULTIMATELY BECOME BIPOLAR

Irritability

Temper tantrums, poor tolerance of frustration

Hyperactivity, impulsivity, increased aggression

By parental report, the cluster of above symptoms may characterize the earliest precursors to an illness eventually associated with more classic mania

FEATURES UNIQUE TO YOUTH IN BIPOLAR ILLNESS

Protracted episodes

Mixed episode

Rapid cycling

High risk for suicide

ASSESSMENT

Corroborate data from patient, parent, and school

Chronic affective/psychotic symptoms

Understanding pre-morbidity and comorbidity

Rule out medical cause of manic episodes

Rule out neurodevelopmental abnormalities

Assess psychosocial functions/determine stress

Assess academic performance

Understand the family dynamics

DIFFERENTIAL DIAGNOSIS OF BIPOLAR DISORDER

ADHD and conduct disorder

Substance-induced mood disorder

Medical condition, e.g., hyperthyroidism, head trauma, multiple sclerosis

Schizophrenia

Anxiety disorder

Autistic spectrum disorder

AVAILABLE TREATMENT OF BIPOLAR DISORDER

Mood stabilizer: lithium, valproic acid, lamotrigine, carbamazepine, gabapentin, topiramate

Atypical antipsychotic: olanzapine, risperidone, quetiapine, aripiprazole, clozapine

Others typical antipsychotics

Antidepressants: SSRIs, fluoxetine, citalopram, sertraline, fluvoxamine

Newer: venlafaxine, bupropion, mirtazapine

Benzodiazepine

ECT

Lithium: data limited; adult guidelines being used. Non-response due to mixed/rapid cycling mood disorder-comorbidity. Noncompliance with lithium due to side effects—acne, weight gain, tremor—may limit the use. Cognitive side effects are not increased.

Valproic acid/carbamazepine: well tolerated in adolescent population. Good results in mixed states and rapid cyclers. Side effects: polycystic disease of ovary, hair loss

TREATMENT OF MANIA

Mania + non-psychotic: Atypical antipsychotic +/- mood stabilizer

Mania + psychotic: Atypical antipsychotic + mood stabilizer

Mania + psychosis + partial or no-response: Atypical antipsychotic + mood stabilizer

MANAGEMENT OF MIXED, MANIC AND RAPID CYCLIC MOOD DISORDER

Combination of anti-manic agents

Avoid antidepressant

Avoid psychostimulants

Rule out medical causes such as thyroid disease

Rule out substance abuse

BIPOLAR DISORDER—DEPRESSION

Check thyroid function

Maximize current mood stabilization

Atypical antipsychotics

Lithium vs. lamotrigine

Antidepressants: SSRI

TREATMENT RESISTANCE ISSUES

Find out the reasons for non-compliance:
- Denial of the illness
- Lack of education
- Striving for independence
- Conflicts with parents
- Conflicts within themselves around their peer group

ENHANCING COMPLIANCE

Address self-esteem issues

Address the fear of recurrence

Educate about the illness: mood chart, warning signs, triggers

Convince parents to step out of the struggle by developing trust and providing responsibility

Corroborate with the patient

Support and educate the patient

TREATMENT STRATEGY: MOVING BEYOND EPISODES

Target treatment to the overall burden of illness

Focus on residual symptoms

Consider combination if monotherapy fails

All medications require monitoring

Stress management and sleep hygiene

Diet, caffeine intake, weight watch, healthy lifestyle

PSYCHOSOCIAL MANAGEMENT

Modification of the school program

Psychoeducation to the child and family

Support group: child and adolescent bipolar foundation (CABF): www.bpkids.org

PEDIATRIC BIPOLAR: OUTCOMES

Prepubertal: At 4 years more than 50% have recovered, but over one-third of the time is spent in manic/hypomanic phase.

Adolescent: 96% 5-year recovery, 44% relapse; 100% 1-year recovery, 67% 2-year relapse

Mixed episodes and rapid cycling predict worse outcome

Ten times greater risk of suicide

CONCLUSION

Bipolar disorder can and does occur in childhood and adolescence. Children at risk for early-onset bipolar disorder can be identified. Early diagnosis and treatment of bipolar disorder in children and adolescents may prevent substance abuse, suicide, and other adverse outcomes. Medications commonly used to treat bipolar disorder may not be safe or effective for children and adolescents, yet the consequences of not treating are significant. Psychosocial treatment helps to understand the illness, decrease tension in the family, increase therapeutic alliance and prevent relapse.

REFERENCES

Ahmed, A. B. M. (2000). Handbook of practical psychiatry, 1st Ed. ISBN No. B-984-8170-27-8

American Psychiatric Association. (2013). Diagnostic and statistical manual of mental disorders (5th ed.). Arlington, VA, US: American Psychiatric Publishing, Inc.

Carlson, G. A. (2012). Differential diagnosis of bipolar disorder in children and adolescents. *World Psychiatry, 11*(3), 146–152.

Geller, B., Williams, M., Zimerman, B., Frazier, J., Beringer, L. & Warner, K. L. (1998). Prepubertal and early adolescent bipolarity differentiate from ADHD by manic symptoms, grandiose delusions, ultra-rapid or ultradian cycling. *Journal of Affective Disorders, 51*(2), 81–91.

Klerman, G. L. (1981). Primary Bipolar Subtypes. *Psychiatric Annals, 17.*

Lewis, M. (Ed.). (2002). Child and adolescent psychiatry: A comprehensive textbook (3rd ed.). Philadelphia, PA, US: Lippincott Williams & Wilkins Publishers.

Pfeifer, J. C., Kowatch, R. A., & DelBello, M. P. (2010). Pharmacotherapy of bipolar disorder in children and adolescents: recent progress. *CNS Drugs, 24,* 575.

Sadock, B. J. (2003). *Kaplan & Sadock's Synopsis of Psychiatry* (9th ed.). B. J. Sadock & V. A. Sadock (Eds.). Philadelphia, Pennsylvania, United States: Lippincott Williams & Wilkins.

14. FIRST-EPISODE PSYCHOSIS

OBJECTIVES

This chapter will discuss definitions of first-episode psychosis, goals of early detection and intervention, prodromal features, and early warning signs. Symptoms of psychosis, differential diagnosis, first-episode schizophrenia versus mania spectrum, and assessment and comprehensive treatment of first-episode psychosis will be covered. Treatment challenges of first-episode psychosis, identification of non-adherence in treatment, and medication-related factors for noncompliance will be highlighted. The predictors of clinical and functional outcomes and the prevention of the progression of the disease and improving the outcome will be discussed.

INTRODUCTION

Early treatment close to the onset of illness improves the prognosis of first-episode psychosis. Early detection of high-risk individuals is the first step in their treatment. Longer duration of psychosis is directly associated with poorer outcomes and treatment resistance.

DEFINITION OF FIRST-EPISODE PSYCHOSIS

A severely disturbed mental state involving disorganization of thinking, behaviour, and impaired reality testing ability.

Psychotic symptoms persist for greater than one week without significant improvement.

Psychotic symptoms not explained by a medical disorder or intoxication.

May be associated with substance abuse but not as a direct consequence of substance abuse.

May include non-affective (schizophrenia spectrum) or affective psychosis (mood disorder spectrum).

FACTS ABOUT PSYCHOSIS

Most severe mental disorder (2% to 3% lifetime risk); incidence around 25–30 per 100,000 per year (including affective psychosis).

Most cases have their onset before age 25 and nearly 25% before age 18.

Early signs of psychiatric symptoms and functional problems (prodromal) begin usually in early adolescence.

GOALS OF EARLY DETECTION AND INTERVENTION

To identify individuals at high risk for psychotic illness before illness starts

To identify those at the earliest stage of psychosis

To prevent delay or minimize the severity of florid psychosis

To decrease disability and dysfunction

To limit social withdrawal and isolation

To decrease the risk of comorbid depression and suicide

PRODROMAL FEATURES

Basic features: disturbance in thought and sense of reality

Decreased role functioning

Behavioural problems

Communication problems
Attenuated positive features

EARLY WARNING SIGN OF FIRST-EPISODE PSYCHOSIS

Confusion about what is real or imaginary
Paranoia or suspicion
Exaggerated self-opinion
Heightened or dulled perceptions
Odd thoughts or speech
Loss of friends and intimacy
Passive, unusual, or blunted interests
Blunted or inappropriate emotions
Academic or occupational difficulties

SYMPTOMS OF PSYCHOSIS

Positive symptoms: delusions, hallucinations, disorganized speech (thought process), grossly disorganized behaviour

Negative symptoms: flat affect, paucity of speech, avolition

DIFFERENTIAL DIAGNOSIS OF FIRST-EPISODE PSYCHOSIS

Schizophrenia
Brief psychotic disorder
Schizophreniform disorder
Delusional disorder
Schizoaffective disorder

Affective psychosis (bipolar disorder or major depressive disorder with psychotic features)

Personality disorders (schizotypal, schizoid, paranoid, borderline)

Substance-induced psychotic disorders: suspect psychosis is not substance-induced if symptoms persist greater than 1 month, symptoms are substantially in excess, and if there is a history of non-substance related episodes.

Substance use is a frequent trigger of primary psychiatric illness; frequently "unmasks" an underlying illness; may lower the age of onset.

Substance use may be the result rather than the cause of psychosis.

Psychotic disorder due to general medical condition, e.g., delirium.

Pervasive developmental disorder or other developmental disorder.

Anxiety disorder, somatoform disorder, dissociative disorder, factitious disorder.

Psychosis "not otherwise specified" is a very common diagnosis in children and adolescents. It reveals the limitations of our classification systems. There have been various attempts to classify these patients. Antecedent or prodrome in some and "partial penetrance" or genetic variant in others.

ASSESSMENT OF FIRST-EPISODE PSYCHOSIS

Good history including collateral

Mental status observations

Admit to hospital if necessary

Medical consultation/neurology assessment

Lab investigations

Psychometric/neuropsychological assessment if available

COMPREHENSIVE TREATMENT OF FIRST-EPISODE PSYCHOSIS

Antipsychotics

Psychoeducation

Support and social-skills groups

Occupational therapy

Vocational therapy

Comorbid condition assessments

Cognitive strategies

Substance-abuse counselling

Recreational assessment and rehabilitation

SIMPLIFICATION OF TREATMENT REGIMES

Simple regimes enhance adherence

Create a strong therapeutic alliance with the patient

Educate family and patient

Choose medications with low potential for side effects

FIRST-EPISODE DOSING OF ANTIPSYCHOTICS

"Start Low and Go Slow" towards target dose

Risperidone: 0.5 mg to 4 mg/day

Olanzapine: 5 mg to 15 mg/day

Quetiapine: 200 mg to 800 mg/day

Ziprasidone: 20 mg to 80 mg/day

Aripiprazole: 10 mg to 30 mg/day

Clozapine: 300 mg to 450 mg/day. Rarely used in children/adolescents.

PSYCHOSOCIAL MANAGEMENT

Regular outpatient follow-up, meet with patient alone and with parent

Supportive psychotherapy to deal with any educational/vocational/financial/social needs

Rapport and trust are central

Family support and education: they may need help reducing stressful interactions—"High express emotion"—risk of relapse

Monitor compliance. Look for substance-abuse potential.

Monitor risk of deliberate harm to self and others.

ISSUES OF TREATMENT ADHERENCE IN FIRST-EPISODE PSYCHOSIS

High potential for relapse for those who are non-adherent to their treatment schedule.

Non-adherence is a major risk factor for relapse. Fifty-nine percent of first-episode psychotic patients are partially or completely non-adherent in one year. Thirty-three percent of them are inadequately adherent.

Most common reasons are lack of insight and intolerable side effects of medications.

Adherence declines early after discharge from hospital and increases over time.

IDENTIFICATION OF NON-ADHERENCE IN TREATMENT

Lack of insight and denial of illness

Substance abuse and poor choices

Medication impacts on lifestyle

Obesity is a growing concern

Cognitive impairment and disorganization

Healthcare beliefs

Cultural differences

Stigma and beliefs

Non-adherence in the past

Poor caregiver and social support

Financial costs

MEDICATION-RELATED FACTORS FOR NONCOMPLIANCE

Intolerable side effects of medication, e.g., cognitive blunting, weight gain

High doses

Complicated dose schedule

Multiple medications often mean multiple side effects

Overly sedated

A comprehensive book on the benefits of polypharmacy still needs to be written

FUNCTIONAL RECOVERY FROM FIRST-EPISODE PSYCHOSIS

Recovery is defined as remission of both positive and negative symptoms in addition to an adequate level of social and vocational functioning.

Forty-seven percent of patients achieved full remission of symptoms after 5 years; 25.5% achieved "adequate social functioning" after 2 years. Only 13.7% met full recovery after 5 years.

Better cognitive functioning at the time of stabilization is associated with a full recovery.

Shorter duration of illness predicted recovery and symptom relief.

WHAT PREDICTS CLINICAL AND FUNCTIONAL OUTCOME?

Pre-morbid functioning

Age of onset

Acute versus insidious onset

Shorter duration of untreated psychosis

Delay in treatment

Adherence in treatment

PREVENTING PROGRESSION OF DISEASE AND IMPROVING OUTCOME

Better management of childhood psychotic disorders

Specialized treatment

Special attention to recovery, reintegration, and stigma

Patient and family involvement in collaboration with a service provider

Reducing stress

Making treatment attractive

CONCLUSION

First-episode psychosis is more treatable the closer it is detected to the onset of the illness. Awareness is the key to early intervention. Early detection for high-risk individuals is the first step in their treatment. Quick and easy access to care and reducing delay is pivotal to effecting a change. Adherence is key to symptom remission and functional recovery.

REFERENCES

American Psychiatric Association. (2013). Diagnostic and statistical manual of mental disorders (5th ed.). Arlington, VA, US: American Psychiatric Publishing, Inc.

Epstein, I. (2008). Improving adherence in the first episode psychosis-what is the evidence? Grand Rounds. Brampton Civic Hospital, Brampton, Ontario, Canada.

Lewis, R. (2004). Current approach to the assessment & treatment of adolescent psychosis. Grand Rounds. Brampton Civic Hospital, Brampton, Ontario, Canada.

Malla, A. K., Norman, R. M. G. & Joober, R. (2005). First-Episode Psychosis, Early Intervention, and Outcome: What Have We Learned? *The Canadian Journal of Psychiatry, 50*(14).

15. EATING DISORDERS

OBJECTIVES

This chapter will discuss the clinical presentation of anorexia and bulimia nervosa. Assessment, diagnosis, associated features, comorbidity, medical assessment, and general treatment principles of eating disorders will be discussed. Treatment setting, nutritional rehabilitation, medication management and psychotherapy will be described. Risk identification, prognosis, and relapse prevention will be covered.

INTRODUCTION

Patients with eating disorders display a broad range of symptoms that frequently occur along a continuum. Weight and shape preoccupation and excessive self-evaluation based on weight and shape are the primary symptoms for all eating disorders.

ANOREXIA NERVOSA

Anorexia nervosa (AN) is characterized by a profound disturbance of body image and a relentless pursuit of thinness, often to the point of starvation. The disorder has been recognized for many decades. It is much more prevalent in females than in males and usually has its onset in adolescence. The psychological disturbance in young women within the disorder includes conflicts surrounding the transition from being a girl to a woman, feelings of helplessness, and difficulty in establishing autonomy.

EPIDEMIOLOGY OF ANOREXIA NERVOSA

Although the disorder was initially reported most often among the upper classes, recent epidemiological surveys do not show that distribution.

AN has been reported more frequently over the past several decades with increasing reports of the disorder in prepubertal girls and in males.

Most common ages of onset of AN are the mid-teenage years.

AN is estimated to occur in about 0.5% to 1% of adolescent girls. AN occurs 10 to 20 times more often in females than in males.

DSM-5 CRITERIA FOR ANOREXIA NERVOSA

Refusal to maintain body weight at or above a minimally normal weight for height and age.

An intense fear of gaining weight or becoming fat even though underweight.

Disturbance in the way in which one's body weight or shape is experienced, undue influence of body weight or shape on self-evaluation, or the denial of the seriousness of the current low body weight.

ANOREXIA NERVOSA SUBTYPES

Restricting subtypes: not regularly engaged in bingeing or purging in the last 3 months

Binge eating/purging subtype: regularly engaging in bingeing or purging behaviours in the last 3 months

ASSOCIATED FEATURES

Perfectionism

Obsessive-compulsive personality traits

Rigid, inhibited, harm-avoidant, emotional restraint

Need for exactness, conformity to authority, and difficulty with transitions

Sexual disinterest

Family history of depression, eating disorder, and/or obsessive-compulsive personality disorder

RISK FACTORS

The risks to long-term effect on physical health include:

    A) Growth retardation

    B) Delayed or arrested puberty

    C) Reduced bone density

    D) Higher likelihood of low-birth-weight baby

Risk factors for a poorer outcome:

    A) Excessive weight loss

    B) Vomiting and purging as part of the clinical picture

    C) Poor social adjustment

    D) Poor parental relationships

    E) Male gender

    F) Chronic course of illness

BULIMIA NERVOSA (BN)

BN consists of recurrent episodes of bingeing and purging followed by feelings of guilt and self-disgust.

BN is more prevalent than AN. Estimates of BN range from 1% to 3% of young women. BN is significantly more common in females than in males and onset is often later in adolescence.

Families of BN are less close and more conflictual. Patients find difficulty in controlling their impulses and are often manifested by substance dependence and self-destructive behaviours.

DSM-5 CRITERIA FOR BN

Recurrent episodes of binge eating, which is characterized by both of the following:

    A) Eating a large amount of food in a short period of time, and

    B) Sense of lack of control

Recurrent inappropriate compensatory behaviour in order to prevent weight gain, such as self-induced vomiting, misuse of laxatives, diuretics, enemas, medications, fasting, or excessive exercise.

Binge eating and inappropriate compensatory behaviours both occur on average at least once a week for 3 months.

Self-evaluation is unduly influenced by body weight and shape.

Disturbances do not occur exclusively during the course of anorexia nervosa.

ASSOCIATED FEATURES

More likely to recognize their disorder

Binge eating is often triggered by dysphoric moods, interpersonal stressors, poor body image, or eating a small amount of forbidden food

Novelty-seeking, outgoing, more concerned about sexual attractiveness, impulsive, labile mood, affect dysregulation

More associated with self-harm, substance abuse and cluster B traits

Between binges, bulimic patients typically restrict and diet to the extreme

Family history of obesity, bulimia nervosa, depression, and substance abuse

BINGE EATING DISORDER

A) Recurrent episodes of binge eating characterized by eating in a discrete period of time and sense of lack of control overeating

B) Binge eating episodes are associated with three or more of the following:

1) Eating rapidly
2) Eating until feeling uncomfortably full
3) Eating a large amount of food when not feeling hungry
4) Eating alone in fear of embarrassment by how much one is eating
5) Feeling guilty/depressed afterward

C) Marked distress regarding binge eating is present

D) Binge eating occurs at least once a week for 3 months

E) Binge-eating is not associated with AN or BN

OBESITY

Not an eating disorder

A heterogeneous metabolic disturbance

The vast majority of obese people do not have disturbed eating behaviour or any characteristic psychopathology

COMORBIDITY IN EATING DISORDERS

It is very important to do a full psychiatric assessment as comorbidity is the rule rather than the exception.

Often have multiple impairments in many aspects of their lives.

Important to do a full assessment: past medical history, family dynamics, and past personal history.

	AN	BN
Depression/dysthymia	50%–75%	50%–60%
OCD	15%–20%	
Bipolar disorder		5%–10%
Substance abuse	10%–15%	30%–35%
Anxiety disorders	Social anxiety disorder	PTSD
Personality disorders	Obsessive-compulsive personality disorder (OCPD)	Borderline personality disorder (BD)/ Histrionic personality disorder (HPD)/ Narcissistic personality disorder (NPD) 30%–50%

MEDICAL ASSESSMENT

Need to collaborate with other health professionals

Need ongoing monitoring and assessment of patient's psychiatric and medical status

Need a full physical exam with vitals, height, weight, and dental exam

LABORATORY TESTS

CBC, electrolytes, creatinine, urea, HCO_3, LFT's, calcium, magnesium, phosphate, amylase, protein, glucose, thyroid, and CK

ECG

Bone mineral density

Frequency of checkups and repetition of exams depends on the severity of illness and results of initial tests

Laboratory test results in eating disorders:

- Vomiting: increased amylase, increased bicarbonate, decreased potassium, and decreased chloride with a metabolic alkalosis
- Laxative abuse: metabolic acidosis with decreased potassium and decreased bicarbonate

MULTIMODAL TREATMENT OF EATING DISORDERS

Psychoeducation of parents and youth about the nature of the illness and necessity of intensive treatment.

Determine the level of care (inpatient, day hospital, outpatient treatment) that is appropriate depending on the severity of the disorder and medical compromise.

Set behavioural goals for improving medical and nutritional status.

Re-establish eating as a process based on hunger and satiety cues as well as nourishment.

Supportive psychotherapy, rapport, trust-building, and cognitive behavioural treatment to help develop adaptive cognitive techniques for addressing the distortions regarding weight and body image.

Family therapy: Working with the family is crucial to the success of treatment.

Specific skills-building regarding the development of a balanced lifestyle, including work, play, and social relationships.

School interventions may be required to decrease anxiety for perfectionistic re-doing of homework and maintaining appropriate academic progress.

MEDICATIONS

There are no medications specifically targeting eating disorders.

First line: SSRIs (selective serotonin reuptake inhibitors) for treatment of obsessiveness, depression, and may help in reducing the risk of relapse.

Second line: Atypical antipsychotics: risperidone, olanzapine may be used to facilitate weight gain in the anorexic patient by reducing anxiety, thought distortions, and increasing appetite.

Other medications as appropriate for targeted symptoms and comorbid conditions.

RELAPSE PREVENTION

Recovery is a long, difficult journey but it is possible.

Continue to stress the risk of dieting.

Consolidate improvements and continue to change eating disorder thoughts.

Integrating back into work, school life, relationship, and family.

Continue to look at underlying issues, e.g., low self-esteem.

Expect occasional setbacks under times of stress and look at the triggers.

Make up a written safety plan.

Stick to the goals.

PROGNOSIS FOR AN AND BN

Some cases of AN in children and adolescents are mild and resolve without intensive treatment, however, many will go into adult services with chronic eating problems.

Long-term outcomes for AN generally accept that a third will recover fully, a third will make a partial recovery and a third will have chronic symptoms.

Full recovery may occur in up to 50% and partial recovery in 60%–75% of bulimic patients at a 10-year follow up. Longer follow up leads to lower relapse rates.

CONCLUSION

Anorexia and bulimia nervosa are serious psychiatric disorders that may carry a significant risk of morbidity and mortality. Both conditions need intensely coordinated biopsychosocial management. Risks to physical and emotional health are greater without early intervention, multimodal treatment and long-term follow up. The outcome of anorexia nervosa is poorer than bulimia nervosa.

REFERENCES

American Psychiatric Association. (2013). Diagnostic and statistical manual of mental disorders (5th ed.). Arlington, VA, US: American Psychiatric Publishing, Inc.

Coghill, D., Graham, J., & Bonnar, S., et al. (2009). *Child and Adolescent Psychiatry*. Oxford, United Kingdom: Oxford University Press.

Staab, R., Toronto General Hospital, University Health Network. (January 2018). Grand Rounds presentation, Toronto General Hospital, Toronto, Ontario.

Stubbe, D. (2007). *Child and Adolescent Psychiatry*. Philadelphia, Pennsylvania, United States: Lippincott Williams & Wilkins.

16. PICA

OBJECTIVES

In this chapter, diagnostic criteria, prevalence, course, complications, culture-related diagnostic issues, differential diagnosis, comorbidity, and treatment of pica will be described.

DIAGNOSTIC CRITERIA

Pica is the eating of non-nutritive, non-food substances on a persistent basis for at least one month. This behaviour is inappropriate to the developmental level of the child and not part of a culturally sanctioned practice.

PREVALENCE

Unclear; higher rates in children with intellectual disabilities and autism spectrum disorder

COURSE

Childhood-onset is most commonly reported; however, pica may occur in adolescence and adulthood.

Vitamin deficiency has been postulated as a cause. In a minority of cases, a mineral deficiency (zinc) has been reported.

The most serious complications of pica are lead poisoning from eating paint chips, mechanical bowel obstruction from eating hair or other non-digestible items, and toxoplasmosis or other parasites from eating feces or dirt.

RISK AND PROGNOSTIC FACTORS

Poverty, neglect, lack of supervision, and developmental delay can increase the risk for this condition.

CULTURE-RELATED DIAGNOSTIC ISSUES

In some cultures, the eating of earth or other non-nutritive substances is believed to be of spiritual, medicinal or other social value, or may be culturally supportive or a socially normative practice. Such behaviour does not warrant a diagnosis of pica.

DIAGNOSTIC MARKERS

Abdominal x-ray, ultrasound, and other scanning methods may reveal obstruction related to pica. Blood and other laboratory tests may detect lead poisoning or the nature of the infection.

DIFFERENTIAL DIAGNOSIS

Autism spectrum disorder, schizophrenia, Kleine-Levin syndrome, anorexia nervosa, factitious disorder, and non-suicidal injury

COMORBIDITY

Commonly comorbid with autism spectrum disorder and intellectual disability, and to a lesser degree, schizophrenia and obsessive-compulsive disorder

Other associations with trichotillomania and excoriation disorder

TREATMENT

No specific treatment for pica. An effort should be made to ameliorate any significant psychosocial stressors that are present. If lead is present, the child should be moved to new surroundings. Behavioural techniques, e.g., mild aversion therapy or negative reinforcement. Increasing parental attention may have positive results. In some patients, correction of iron or zinc deficiency has resulted in the elimination of pica. Medical /surgical complications that develop secondarily to the pica must also be treated.

CONCLUSION

Pica is the eating of non-food substances, which may lead to serious medical complications. Prevalence is unclear. Culture-related diagnostic issues need to be considered. Comorbidities have to be identified. No specific treatment is available. Attention has to be given to stressors with behavioural techniques and medical management.

REFERENCES

American Psychiatric Association. (2013). Diagnostic and statistical manual of mental disorders (5th ed.). Arlington, VA, US: American Psychiatric Publishing, Inc.

17. RUMINATION DISORDER

OBJECTIVES
Definitions, epidemiology, course, risk factors, associated features, differential diagnosis, treatment and outcome will be discussed in this chapter.

DEFINITION
Repeated regurgitation of food over a period of at least one month. Regurgitated food may be re-chewed, re-swallowed, or spit out. It is not attributable to a gastrointestinal condition.

EPIDEMIOLOGY
Prevalence data is inconclusive. Commonly occurs in individuals with intellectual disabilities.

ETIOLOGY
Unknown

DEVELOPMENT AND COURSE
Onset can occur in infancy, childhood, adolescence, or adulthood. Severe malnutrition can potentially be fatal in infancy.

RISK FACTORS

Lack of stimulation, neglect, stressful life situations, and problematic parent-child relationship

ASSOCIATED FEATURES

Infants with rumination disorder display a characteristic position of straining and arching the back with the head held back, making sucking movements with their tongue. Weight loss and failure to make expected weight gains are common features in infants with rumination disorder.

DIFFERENTIAL DIAGNOSIS

Gastrointestinal disorder

TREATMENT

Psychotherapy for parents, parent training, positive attention and interaction

Aversion conditioning involving a mild electric shock or squirting an unpleasant substance in the child's mouth whenever rumination occurs

Behavioural techniques: aversive conditioning

Any concomitant medical complications must also be treated

OUTCOME

Little is known of the outcome, but it ranges from spontaneous remission, to malnutrition, to failure to thrive, to death.

CONCLUSION

Rumination disorder is the repeated regurgitation of food. Epidemiology is inconclusive and etiology is unknown. Onset may occur within infancy to adulthood. Aversion therapy may help. Little is known regarding the outcome.

REFERENCES

American Psychiatric Association. (2013). Diagnostic and statistical manual of mental disorders (5th ed.). Arlington, VA, US: American Psychiatric Publishing, Inc.

Sadock, B. J. (2003). *Kaplan & Sadock's Synopsis of Psychiatry* (9th ed.). B. J. Sadock & V. A. Sadock (Eds.). Philadelphia, Pennsylvania, United States: Lippincott Williams & Wilkins.

18. ENCOPRESIS

OBJECTIVES
In this chapter, the definition of encopresis, as well as the types, epidemiology, etiology, clinical features, assessment, differential diagnosis and management of encopresis will be described.

DEFINITION
Encopresis is the repeated intentional or involuntary fecal soiling in clothing or inappropriate places at least once monthly for at least 3 months in a child that is 4 years of age or older when full bowel control is expected.

TYPES
With constipation and overflow incontinence

Without constipation and overflow incontinence

EPIDEMIOLOGY
An estimated 1% of 5-year-olds suffer from encopresis. Boys are 2.5 to 6 times more commonly affected than girls. Children with lower cognitive functioning and lower socioeconomic status tend to have higher rates of encopresis.

Children with encopresis often respond positively to the treatment of constipation.

ETIOLOGY

Child who has toilet-related fears

Inadequate or punitive toilet training

Constipation that makes defecating painful

Due to severe constipation, colon (lower intestine) becomes loaded with feces and distended like a balloon (megacolon).

Ultimately colon loses sensation for bowel movement and liquid stool leaks around impacted stools and the child is unaware and unable to exert control. Stress-induced diarrhea may induce encopresis.

Without constipation, encopresis is the deliberate soiling in inappropriate places. Child experiences extreme distress that he/she is unable to communicate directly (e.g., anger, fear of abuse).

ASSESSMENT

A joint approach involving the pediatrician, child psychiatrist and primary-care team needs to be part of the assessment.

The assessment includes complete psychiatric and medical evaluation. The psychiatric evaluation includes assessment for associated disorders. A phobic or anxious child may avoid using the toilet, with soiling when they can no longer hold it.

An ADHD child may not stop to go to the bathroom. An oppositional, angry or abused child may soil willfully.

Mentally retarded children may have difficulty with hygiene and may have difficulty learning to use the toilet appropriately.

A detailed history of bowel function, nature and pattern of soiling, attempts to train or treat, bathroom habits, and environment is needed.

Physical disorders, e.g., Hirschsprung disease or congenital megacolon, irritable bowel disease, thyroid disease, hypercalcemia, lactase deficiency, Spina bifida, rectal stenosis, anal fissure, as well as other neurological disorders have to be ruled out.

MANAGEMENT

With constipation and overflow incontinence type:

- Medical: Laxative and bowel cleanout; stool softeners to prevent constipation; Cisapride is a possible treatment; educate about bowel function and bowel hygiene
- Psychosocial: Relaxation training, regular toileting routine, behavioural management, biofeedback, psychotherapy for associated disorders

Without constipation and overflow incontinence type:

- Medical: No specific medical intervention
- Psychosocial: Behavioural therapy, regular toileting routine, parent-management training, assessment and treatment if abuse or high environmental stress, individual and family therapy

OUTCOME

The majority of children with encopresis who are constipated will do well with correct bowel management. Poor prognosis is associated with chronic cases with systemic family or social problems.

CONCLUSION

Encopresis is repeated intentional or involuntary fecal soiling in clothes or inappropriate places. It may be with or without constipation and overflow incontinence. Deliberate soiling in inappropriate places is due to extreme emotional distress. Assessment and management include a complete psychiatric and medical evaluation, regular toileting routine, and high environmental stress reduction. Individual and family therapy are often helpful.

REFERENCES

American Psychiatric Association. (2013). Diagnostic and statistical manual of mental disorders (5th ed.). Arlington, VA, US: American Psychiatric Publishing, Inc.

Coghill, D., Graham, J., & Bonnar, S., et al. (2009). *Child and Adolescent Psychiatry*. Oxford, United Kingdom: Oxford University Press.

Stubbe, D. (2007). *Child and Adolescent Psychiatry*. Philadelphia, Pennsylvania, United States: Lippincott Williams & Wilkins.

19. ENURESIS

OBJECTIVES

The definition of enuresis, as well as the types, epidemiology, etiology, and management of enuresis will be described in this chapter.

DEFINITION

Enuresis is the repeated intentional or involuntary voiding of urine during the day or night at least twice a week for at least 3 months, causing functional impairment and at an age of at least 5 years old.

Most children achieve daytime bladder control 1–2 years prior to nighttime control. It is unusual for a child to display daytime enuresis without nocturnal enuresis.

TYPES OF ENURESIS

Primary (never dry)

Secondary (follows a period of continence)

Nocturnal

Diurnal (daytime)

Both

EPIDEMIOLOGY

An estimated 5% to10% of 5-year-olds and around 3% to 5% of 10-year-olds suffer from enuresis. This rate decreases to 1% by adolescence and adulthood. Boys display more primary enuresis than girls. For both boys and girls, there is a spontaneous decline of 5% to 10% of cases per year. Secondary enuresis has a similar incidence in boys and girls. Nocturnal enuresis: more common in boys after age 5.

ETIOLOGY

Primary causes:

- Idiopathic
- Familial

Secondary causes:

- Urinary tract infection
- Constipation
- Stressful life events
- ADHD
- Structural abnormality such as spina bifida occulta
- Diurnal enuresis: more common in girls after age 5 years
- Over-absorption in play and or leaving it too late
- Small/irritable bladder
- Pelvic floor insufficiency

ASSESSMENT

Initial medical evaluation is required to rule out medical causes. Family history should concentrate on other family members with a history of enuresis, as well as a family history of diabetes and renal disease. Psychiatric evaluation should concentrate on the assessment of associated psychiatric symptoms (especially anxiety and ADHD) and recent psychosocial stressors and trauma.

MANAGEMENT

Nocturnal enuresis:

- Education and reassurance: The problem is common, often familial, frequently self-limiting, and not intentional. This may be all that is required in preschoolers.
- Practical advice: Reduce evening fluid intake, lift to the toilet at parental bedtime, use mattress covers, avoidance of pull-up nappies (which can prolong the problem)
- Behavioural: Reduce punishment, increase positive reinforcement, star charts, token rewards, etc.
- Alarms: Pad and buzzer; this consists of a sensor in the pants that sounds an alarm when wet. This conditions the child to connect the urge to void with the signal to wake.
- Medication: Oral or intranasal desmopressin (antidiuretic hormone analogue). This allows a short dryness period that enables attendance at camp/sleepovers, etc. Tricyclic antidepressants are effective at reducing wetting (secondary to antimuscarinic effect) and are used occasionally in older children/adolescents.

Diurnal enuresis:

- Behavioural: Regular visit to the toilet, positive reinforcement
- Physical: Bladder training—learning to drink increasing amounts and holding on for an increasing amount of time, pelvic floor exercises

CONCLUSION

Enuresis is the repeated intentional or involuntary voiding of urine during the day or at night. This is a relatively common condition and may occur due to medical or emotional reasons. Complete psychiatric and medical evaluation is required. Medical intervention complemented with behavioural management is effective.

REFERENCES

American Psychiatric Association. (2013). Diagnostic and statistical manual of mental disorders (5th ed.). Arlington, VA, US: American Psychiatric Publishing, Inc.

Coghill, D., Graham, J., & Bonnar, S., et al. (2009). *Child and Adolescent Psychiatry*. Oxford, United Kingdom: Oxford University Press.

Stubbe, D. (2007). *Child and Adolescent Psychiatry*. Philadelphia, Pennsylvania, United States: Lippincott Williams & Wilkins.

20. OBSESSIVE-COMPULSIVE AND RELATED DISORDERS

OBJECTIVES

In this chapter, obsessive-compulsive disorder (OCD), trichotillomania, body dysmorphic disorder, hoarding disorder, and excoriation will be described.

OBSESSIVE-COMPULSIVE DISORDER

Definition

Obsessive-compulsive disorder is characterized by recurrent, time-consuming obsessions or compulsive behaviours that cause distress and/or impairment.

Epidemiology

Lifetime prevalence rates of 2% to 3%

Monozygotic twins 75%, dizygotic twins 32%

Ten percent of children with OCD may have the symptoms precipitated by pediatric autoimmune neuropsychiatric disorders associated with streptococcal infections (PANDAS)

Diagnosis

Either obsessions or compulsions

Obsessions:

- Not (simply) excessive worry about real-life problems
- Attempts made to ignore/neutralize obsession with other thoughts or actions
- Patient aware obsessions originate from own mind and are not thought insertions, etc.

Compulsions:

- Drive to perform repetitive behaviours (washing, ordering, checking) or mental acts (praying, counting, word repetition) in response to obsessions or in keeping with rigidly applied rules
- Carried out with the goal of reducing distress, preventing dreaded event/situation although no realistic connection between compulsion and anticipated outcome

Recognition that obsessions or compulsions are excessive or unreasonable (not applicable in younger children)

Obsessions or compulsions cause distress, are time-consuming, or interfere with normal functioning

Treatment

Cognitive behavioural therapy (CBT)

SSRI, Clomipramine

Prognosis

Tends to be refractory and chronic

Conclusion

OCD is recurrent obsessions and compulsions and tends to be chronic in nature with significant psychosocial impairment. Medication in conjunction with cognitive behavioural therapy decreases symptoms of OCD.

TRICHOTILLOMANIA

Diagnostic Criteria

Recurrent pulling out of one's hair resulting in hair loss, with repeated attempts to decrease or stop hair pulling

Hair pulling causes significant distress or impairment in social, occupational, or other important areas of functioning

Clinical Presentation

Trichotillomania patients may experience an increasing sense of tension and achieve a sense of release or gratification from pulling out their hair. Hair pulling may occur from any region of the body in which hair grows. Most common sites are scalp, eyebrows, and eyelids. Hair pulling may occur in brief episodes scattered throughout the day. Patterns of hair loss are highly variable. Areas of complete alopecia, as well as areas of thinned hair density, are common. The individual may attempt to conceal or camouflage hair loss by using makeup, scarves, or wigs.

Prevalence

Prevalence for adolescents and adults is 1% to 2%. Females are more frequently affected. Trichotillomania generally begins at the onset of puberty. The course is often chronic with waxing and waning if the disorder is untreated. Symptoms may worsen in females. The minority of individuals remits without subsequent relapse within a few years of onset.

Risk Factors

There is evidence for genetic vulnerability. The disorder is more common in individuals with obsessive-compulsive disorder and their first-degree relatives than the general population.

Culture-Related Issues

Trichotillomania appears to manifest similarly across cultures, although there is a paucity of data from non-Western regions.

Diagnosis

Most individuals with trichotillomania admit to hair pulling. However, skin biopsy and dermoscopy differentiate the disorder from other causes of alopecia. Dermoscopy shows a range of characteristic features, including decreased hair density, short vellus hair, and broken hairs with different shaft lengths.

Differential Diagnosis

Normative hair removal/manipulation

Other obsessive-compulsive and related disorders: individuals with OCD may pull out hair as a part of their rituals. An individual with body dysmorphic disorder may pull out hair they perceive as ugly, asymmetrical, or abnormal.

Neurodevelopmental disorder, i.e., stereotypic movement disorder and tic disorder may lead to hair pulling.

Psychotic disorder: individual may remove hair in response to hallucination or delusion

Another medical condition

Substance-related disorder

Comorbidities

Trichotillomania is often accompanied by other mental disorders: most commonly, depression and skin picking (excoriation) and body-focused repetitive behavioural disorder, e.g., nail-biting.

Functional Consequences

Can cause distress as well as social and occupational impairment. May be irreversible damage to hair growth and hair quality. Medical consequences include digit purpura, musculoskeletal injury, blepharitis, and dental damage. Swallowing of hair (trichophagia) may lead to trichobezoars, with anemia, abdominal pain, hematemesis, nausea, vomiting, bowel obstruction and even perforation.

Treatment

Treatment usually involves a psychiatrist and a dermatologist in a joint endeavour. An antidepressant agent may lead to dermatological improvement. A patient who responds poorly to SSRIs, augmentation with pimozide (orap), a dopamine blocker, may lead to improvement. Lithium has been used to decrease impulsivity and mood instability. Behavioural treatment, such as biofeedback, insight-oriented psychotherapy, and hypnotherapy have all been mentioned as effective treatment modalities.

Prognosis

Trichotillomania usually begins in childhood or adolescence. Late onset may be associated with an increased likelihood of chronicity.

Conclusion

A trichotillomanic patient may experience an increasing sense of tension and achieve a sense of release or gratification from pulling out their hair. Trichotillomania is often accompanied by other mental disorders. Antidepressants and various behavioural management techniques have been mentioned as effective treatment modalities.

BODY DYSMORPHIC DISORDER

Definition

Preoccupation with one or more perceived defects in physical appearance that are not observable to others.

The individual may be involved in a repetitive behaviour, such as mirror checking or skin picking in response to the appearance concern.

The person is preoccupied with appearance and this causes significant distress.

HOARDING DISORDER

Definition

Hoarding disorder is characterized by a persistent difficulty in discarding of possessions because of a perceived need to save them. Distress associated with discarding possessions.

The difficulty in discarding possessions results in the accumulation of possessions that congest and clutter in active living areas.

Hoarding causes clinically significant distress or impairment in functioning.

Murad Bakht, FRCP (C)

EXCORIATION (SKIN-PICKING) DISORDER

Definition

Recurrent skin picking resulting in skin lesions

Repeated attempts to decrease or stop skin picking

Skin picking causes clinically significant distress or impairment in functioning

REFERENCES

American Psychiatric Association. (2013). Diagnostic and statistical manual of mental disorders (5th ed.). Arlington, VA, US: American Psychiatric Publishing, Inc.

Coghill, D., Graham, J., & Bonnar, S., et al. (2009). *Child and Adolescent Psychiatry*. Oxford, United Kingdom: Oxford University Press.

Sadock, B. J. (2003). *Kaplan & Sadock's Synopsis of Psychiatry* (9th ed.). B. J. Sadock & V. A. Sadock (Eds.). Philadelphia, Pennsylvania, USA: Lippincott Williams & Wilkins.

Stubbe, D. (2007). *Child and Adolescent Psychiatry*. Philadelphia, Pennsylvania, United States: Lippincott Williams & Wilkins.

University of Toronto. (1998). MCCQE Review notes and Lecture series. Toronto, Canada: Faculty of Medicine, University of Toronto.

21. PRINCIPLES OF PSYCHIATRIC TREATMENT

OBJECTIVES

In this chapter the major classes of medication use in psychiatry, including the therapeutic use of psychostimulants, antidepressants, antipsychotics, mood stabilizers, anxiolytics, and the use of electroconvulsive therapy (ECT) will be described. The various types of psychotherapy used for children and adolescents will be covered as well.

INTRODUCTION

An appropriate treatment plan evolves from a thorough psychiatric evaluation.

Thorough feedback about the results of the evaluation sets the stage for providing treatment recommendations.

A therapeutic alliance must be developed with the patient.

Setting the stage of mutual respect and open communication at the outset of treatment begins an alliance that may be the most powerful therapeutic tool you have.

PSYCHOPHARMACOLOGY

Medication may be an important component of a multimodal treatment plan.

For all psychotropics used there should be a careful consideration of risk and benefit of the treatment.

Rating forms of symptoms prior to and following the initiation of medication may be helpful in qualifying the effectiveness and side effects.

A careful medical and medication/substance history must be taken prior to the initiation of any medication, with laboratory tests, ECG, or other tests as appropriate.

ESSENTIALS FOR THE USE OF PHARMACOTHERAPY

Review the patient's medical history, drug allergies and past drug reaction

Identify treatable symptoms and establish treatment goals

Initiate medications at low doses and assess dosing schedule

Monitor therapy regularly, e.g., side effects, blood pressure, height, weight, etc.

Use rating scale to assess side-effect benefit

Limit and manage side effects; avoid adding medication that may cause drug interactions

Determine treatment duration

Minimize polytherapy

MAJOR CLASSES OF MEDICATIONS USED IN PSYCHIATRY

Stimulants

Stimulant medication acts to enhance dopamine and noradrenergic transmission.

They improve both cognitive and behavioural functioning.

They are considered the first-line medication in the treatment of attention deficit hyperactivity disorder (ADHD).

Stimulant medications come in short- and long-acting preparations.

Most commonly reported side effects are appetite suppression and sleep disturbance.

Less frequently reported side effects are mood disturbance, headache, abdominal pain, and rarely growth retardation.

Common stimulants include methylphenidate and dextroamphetamine such as; Ritalin, Concerta, Biphentin, Foquest, Dexedrine, Adderall XR, Vyvanse.

Antidepressants

Antidepressants comprise four main groups of drugs:
1. Tricyclic antidepressants (TCA)
2. Selective serotonin reuptake inhibitors (SSRI)
3. Newer atypical antidepressants
4. Monoamine oxidase inhibitors (MOAI)

Therapeutic use of Antidepressants

In clinical practice, antidepressants are used for unipolar depression or anxiety.

Antidepressant's effectiveness is expected after 4–6 weeks.

Once the patient achieves remission, the antidepressant should be continued for at least 6–12 months

In recurrent depression, the antidepressant should continue for an indefinite period.

Tricyclic Antidepressants (TCA)

Amitriptyline (Elavil) 25–100mg/day

Imipramine (Tofranil) 25–100mg/day

Nortriptyline (Pamelor) 30–150mg/day

Side effects: orthostatic hypotension, sedation, weight gain, GI intolerance, sexual dysfunction,

Monitoring: EKG, blood pressure, heart rate, weight

Serotonin Reuptake Inhibitors (SSRI)

Citalopram (Celexa)

Escitalopram (Cipralex)

Fluoxetine (Prozac)

Fluvoxamine (Luvox)

Paroxetine (Paxil)

Sertraline (Zoloft)

Side effects: GI intolerance, sexual dysfunction, activation of mania, sleep disturbance

Monitoring: weight, liver function, drug interaction, manic symptoms, suicidality

Atypical Antidepressants

Bupropion

Venlafaxine

Mirtazapine

Side effects: agitation, insomnia, GI intolerance, activation of mania, sleep disturbance, sexual dysfunction, hypertension, weight gain, somnolence

Monitoring: weight, blood pressure, seizure threshold, drug interaction, lipids, liver function

Mood Stabilizers

Three commonly used well-studied mood stabilizers:
1. Lithium: usual dose 600–1800 mg/day in divided dose

    Side effects: sedation, thirst, polydipsia, weight gain, GI intolerance, tremor, hypothyroidism serum level 0.6–1.5 meq/lit

2. Valproate: usual dose 750–3800 mg/day in divided dose

    Side effects: sedation, thrombocytopenia, alopecia, nausea, weight gain, tremor, GI upset, hepatotoxicity, agranulocytosis, neutropenia

    Monitoring: CBC, liver function tests, weight

    Serum level 50–125 micrograms/ml

3. Carbamazepine: usual dose 400–800 mg/day

    Side effects: dizziness, rash, impaired coordination, slurred speech, ataxia, agranulocytosis

    Serum level 4–12 micrograms/ml

Anxiolytics

Drugs with anxiolytic activity include:
- Benzodiazepines, e.g., Alprazolam, Lorazepam, Diazepam
- Buspirone
- TCAs, SSRIs
- Alpha agonists, such as clonidine, or guanfacine
- Beta blockers, e.g., Propanolol

- Benzodiazepines are used in the treatment of acute anxiety, panic, and sleep disturbance, and may be useful for acute treatment of neuroleptic-induced akathisia
- Disadvantages of benzodiazepine are sedation, disinhibition, psychological, and physical dependence

Antipsychotics

There are two classes of antipsychotics used in clinical practice: typical and atypical.

Both categories of antipsychotics effectively treat the hallmarks of psychosis, including hallucinations, delusions, bizarre behaviours, disordered thinking, and severe agitation.

Newer atypical antipsychotics are more successful at ameliorating the negative symptoms such as apathy and avolition. They have fewer side effects, which has led to the establishment of atypical antipsychotics as first-line antipsychotic medication.

Antipsychotic medications are used to treat schizophrenia, depression with psychotic features, bipolar illness, autistic disorders, severe violent behaviour, etc.

Potential side effects of antipsychotics include sedation, neuroleptic malignant syndrome, weight gain, extrapyramidal symptoms (EPS), tardive dyskinesia, hyperprolactinemia, diabetes

Typical antipsychotics: chlorpromazine, haloperidol

Atypical antipsychotics: aripiprazole, risperidone, olanzapine, quetiapine, ziprasidone, clozapine

ELECTROCONVULSIVE THERAPY (ECT)

Induction of grand mal convulsion by means of an externally applied electric stimulus for the treatment of certain mental disorders

Indication: Major depression with high suicide risk, manic phase of bipolar mood disorder, postpartum psychosis, schizophrenia with catatonia or depression

Doses: total number of treatments may range from 6 to 20

Side effects: transient memory loss, post-treatment delirium, headache, muscle pain, prolonged seizure

PSYCHOTHERAPY

Psychotherapy may be defined as the therapy that uses interpersonal interaction between a therapist and a patient in order to improve adaptive functioning and reduce symptoms and distress (Kazdin, 1990).

A trained therapist establishes a professional relationship with a patient for the purpose of removing, modifying or retarding existing symptoms, or attenuating or reversing disturbed patients' behaviour, and of promoting positive personality growth and development.

COMMON TYPES OF PSYCHOTHERAPY

Individual psychotherapy

Group therapy

Family therapy

Recent reviews of the literature have shown that various forms of refined psychotherapeutic interventions do alleviate suffering in children and their families (Kazdin,1990; Kovacs & Lohr, 1995).

SPECIFIC THERAPIES FOR SPECIFIC DISORDERS

Studies have shown that psychoanalytically oriented psychotherapy, cognitive behavioural therapy, and cognitive-problem-solving skills training often associated with parent management training are effective means of therapy for children with a psychiatric disorder.

Dynamic psychotherapies are likely to be effective with internalizing or emotional disorders, e.g., anxiety, depression.

Cognitive therapies combined with parent management training will probably be more effective with externalizing disorders.

1. Psychoanalytically Oriented Psychotherapy

Aim of therapy is to enhance self-awareness or insight in order to resolve conflict, promote adaptive skills, and reduce suffering.

Other forms of psychotherapy such as non-intensive or supportive or brief psychotherapy without the participation of parents may be useful.

2. Cognitive Therapies

In this process, the child develops inner speech which mediates social behaviour.

The therapist instructs the child to "talk and direct himself/herself" to use socially desirable behaviour or to suppress unacceptable behaviours. With the help of the therapist, the child becomes active in the process of understanding self and selecting the most adaptive response among alternatives.

3. Cognitive Behavioural Therapy (CBT)

This is a form of therapy that combines elements of cognitive and behavioural therapy. Children either individually or in a group are instructed through well-defined learning steps to confront anxiety-arousing conditions or consider alternatives before choosing the most adaptive response in social interactions. A review of the literature has shown that CBT is particularly effective for obsessive-compulsive disorder and depressive disorders in children and adolescents.

A group form of CBT, problem-solving skills training (PSST) is promising for children presenting with behavioural disorders. Another variant of PSST in group form therapy is often called "social-skills training."

PARENT MANAGEMENT TRAINING

The therapy addresses a faulty parent(s)-child interaction which is associated with the development and perpetuation of aggressive and oppositional behaviour in children. The aim of parent management training is to train the parents to readdress the faulty interaction between them and their child. A healthy interaction will reinforce appropriate behaviour and suppress inappropriate behaviour. This is promising for an aggressive child but has its limit. Multi-problem families with serious parental pathology and marital disharmony do not respond to parent management training.

CONCLUSION

Medication may be an important component of a multimodal treatment plan. All psychotropics used for children and adolescents should be carefully considered for the risk and benefit of the treatment and polytherapy must be minimized. Appropriate psychotherapy should always be included as part of the treatment modalities.

REFERENCES

Kazdin, A. E. (1990). Psychotherapy for children and adolescents. *Annual Review of Psychology, 41*, 21–54.

Kotsopoulos, S. (1997). Psychotherapies in childhood disorders; An overview of current trends: A: Review course of psychiatry. Ottawa, 1997.

Kovacs, M. & Lohr, W. D. (1995). Research on psychotherapy with children and adolescents: An overview of evolving trends and current issues. *J. Abn. Child Psychology, 23*, 11–30.

Sadock, B. J. (2003). *Kaplan & Sadock's Synopsis of Psychiatry* (9th ed.). B. J. Sadock & V. A. Sadock (Eds.). Philadelphia, Pennsylvania, United States: Lippincott Williams & Wilkins.

Virani, A., Kalyna, Z., Bezchlibny-Butler, J., Jeffries, J., & Procyshyn, R. M. (Eds.). (1994). *Clinical Handbook of Psychotropic Drugs, 19th Revised Edition*. Hogrefe Publishing, Göttingen.

22. CHILD ABUSE AND NEGLECT

OBJECTIVES

This chapter will define various types of child maltreatment, global prevalence, and risk factors for physical, emotional, and sexual abuse. Circumstances of abuse, parental characteristics, and identifying features of abuse and neglect will be explained. The psychological effect of maltreatment in childhood and consequences in adult life will be highlighted. Assessment and management of abuse and domestic violence will be discussed.

INTRODUCTION

Child abuse has become a major public health concern globally. It is associated with significant psychological morbidity in childhood and adolescence and continues throughout the lifespan. Various epidemiological studies support that child abuse and neglect have increased dramatically across the world and are at epidemic proportions. Children and youth are developmentally, psychiatrically, and physically scarred as a result.

DEFINITION OF CHILD MALTREATMENT

Physical abuse

Infliction of non-accidental physical injury to a child, ranging from minor bruises to death, by a caregiver or other individual who is responsible for the child.

Sexual abuse

Any sexual act involving a child that is intended to provide sexual gratification to the caregiver or another individual who has responsibility for the child.

Child neglect

Failure to provide for a child's basic needs:

1) Physical neglect
2) Educational neglect
3) Emotional neglect
4) Medical neglect

Emotional abuse (psychological/verbal/mental abuse)

Parents were not able to protect their children while under their care, either intentionally, such as by an act of neglect, abandonment, or other reasons, or by other caregivers that could cause serious behavioural, cognitive, emotional, or mental disorders.

GLOBAL PREVALENCE OF CHILD MALTREATMENT AND ABUSE

In the USA there were an estimated 900,000 reports of child maltreatment in 2002. Of those, 60% involved child neglect,

20% physical abuse, 10% sexual abuse, and 7% emotional maltreatment. An estimated 1,400 children died of maltreatment in 2002.

Girls are 5 times more likely to be the victim of sexual abuse. Infant boys have the highest rate of fatalities.

One well-conducted large-scale UK study indicated 21% mild forms of physical abuse and 7% severe physical abuse. Six percent admitted serious neglect. Only 1% reported sexual abuse by parents/caregivers.

CANADIAN INCIDENCE REPORT OF CHILD ABUSE

Canadian incidence study (CIS) (2008) of reported child abuse and neglect indicates:

- Rate of child maltreatment investigation was 39.2 per 1000 children
- 36% of the total investigations were substantiated cases of child maltreatment (14.2 per 1000 children)
- Among the substantiated cases, 4.9 per 1000 children (34% cases) had exposure to intimate partner violence (IPV)
- 4.8 per 1000 children for neglect (34% cases)
- 2.9 per 1000 children for physical abuse (20% cases)
- 1.2 per 1000 children for emotional maltreatment (9% cases)
- 0.4 per 1000 children for sexual abuse (3% cases)

PHYSICAL ABUSE

Modes of physical abuse include:
- Hitting/shaking/throwing

- Poisoning
- Burning/scalding
- Suffocating
- Drowning

Sexual abuse:

- May involve forcing a child to take part in sexual activity whether or not the child is aware of what is happening
- May involve physical contact, including penetrative or non-penetrative acts
- May involve non-contact activities, e.g., encouraging a child to behave in sexually inappropriate ways

INDICATOR FOR RISK OF SEXUAL ABUSE

Sexual knowledge and/behaviour that seems inappropriate to a child's age and maturity

Sexual play demonstrating sexual knowledge

Running away and fear of certain adults

Regressive behaviour

Hostility/aggression to others

Sleep and eating disturbances

Disclosures to adults, possibly a partial account

Promiscuity, pregnancy, sexually transmitted infections

EMOTIONAL ABUSE

Definition: persistent emotional maltreatment causing severe and persistent adverse effects on the child's emotional development

Some level of emotional abuse is involved in all types of maltreatment

Conveying to a child that they are worthless/unloved/inadequate

Developmentally inappropriate expectations

Overprotection

Limiting a child's exploration and learning

Failure to provide adequate stimulation

Preventing the child from participating in normal social interaction

Exposing the child to ill-treatment

Causing the child to feel frequently frightened or in danger

Emotionally unavailable parenting

Using the child for the fulfillment of parents' psychological needs is often unrecognized

Victims are unlikely to complain

Its presentation is non-specific

No specific findings on examination

MUNCHAUSEN'S SYNDROME BY PROXY

This rare condition occurs when false evidence of an illness is given by the caregiver in order to mislead the medical profession.

Its presentation pattern includes:

- Fabricating an illness
- Doctor/hospital shopping
- The young child's mother usually makes up the story. Sometimes these mothers are in the healthcare profession.

The warning signs are:

- Recurrent unexplained illness
- Inconsistent investigation results
- Treatment ineffective or not tolerated

- Excessively attentive mother refusing to leave the child
- Lack of concern on the mother's part even though the signs and symptoms are serious

RISK FACTORS FOR CHILD MALTREATMENT

Child factors:

- Premature birth weight, birth anomalies
- Difficult temperament
- Physical/cognitive/emotional disability or chronic illness
- ADHD, aggression, and behavioural problems
- Childhood trauma in a younger child

Family factors:

- Domestic violence
- Poor family communications and problem-solving skills
- Parents having been maltreated as a child
- Highly stressed family: financial stress, single parent, lots of children in the home, low employability, disability
- Parental psychopathology, substance abuse, poor impulse control
- Inaccurate knowledge and expectations about childhood development

Social and environmental factors:

- Low socioeconomic status, homelessness
- Dangerous neighbourhood
- Social isolation and lack of support
- Lack of access to healthcare and childcare

- Poor schools
- Exposure to environmental toxins

INDICATORS FOR RISK OF PHYSICAL ABUSE

Delay or failure to seek help

Vague/inconsistent accounts

Account not compatible with injury

Abnormal parental affect—lack of concern/hostility

Child looks sad, withdrawn, frightened

Child says something suggesting abuse

Bruises or fractures, or fractures in a non-mobile child

PARENTAL CHARACTERISTICS FOR PHYSICAL ABUSE

Insensitive care of child

Lack of awareness of child's need

Harsh punishments

Little encouragement

Poor supervision

Psychiatric problems

Domestic violence

Learning disabilities

Past experiences

Abusive or neglectful upbringing

ABUSE CIRCUMSTANCES

Poor social support

Social isolation

Displacement

Persecution

No respite for child

No helpful partner

No friends

Poor housing

Unemployment/debt

Violent neighbourhood

Personal values

Subculture of violence

Self before child

Tired and irritable

Recent arguments

Alcohol and drug abuse

COMMON SITES FOR ACCIDENTAL INJURY

Applies only to mobile child:
- Forehead
- Nose
- Chin
- Shoulders
- Body spine
- Elbows
- Hand, forearms
- Knee, shins

SITES OF POSSIBLE NON-ACCIDENTAL INJURY

Head injuries, fractures

Black eyes

Ear bruises, tears

Chest, arms, shoulders, and neck bruises

Abdomen

Thighs (bruises or scalds)

Cigarette burns

Twisting fractures

Buttock (bruises or scalds)

PSYCHOSOCIAL IMPACT IN ABUSED CHILDREN

Developmental delay

Cognitive/academic difficulties

School adaptation problems

Disturbed emotional development

Poor self-esteem

Maladaptive coping

Limited problem solving

Social communication skills

Poor relationships and difficulties in maintaining relationships

INDICATORS OF NEGLECT

Dirty clothes/body smelly

Chronic infestation (head lice)

Untreated medical condition(s)

Lack of house rules and supervision

Increased rate of accidents

Wetting and soiling

Failure to learn social rules

Attachment disorders, disorganized attachment

Indiscriminately friendly

Poor peer relationships

Low self-esteem

Developmental delays, e.g., language delay

PARENTAL CHARACTERISTICS FOR NEGLECT

Persistent failure to meet a child's basic physical, psychosocial, health, or developmental needs

Maternal substance abuse during pregnancy

Failure to provide adequate food, clothing, or shelter

Failure to protect a child from physical or emotional harm or danger

Failure to ensure access to appropriate medical care or treatment

Being unresponsive to a child's basic emotional needs

PARENTAL CIRCUMSTANCES OF CHRONIC NEGLECT

May occur across societies

Increased risk if:

- Low socioeconomic status
- Poor social resources
- Living in crime-ridden areas
- History of intra-familial violence
- Caregiver forensic history

- Caregiver poor mental health
- Depression
- Alcohol/illicit substance dependence

CHILD CHARACTERISTICS FOR NEGLECT
Special need
Frequent or high pitch cry
Difficult temperament
Weak attachment to the child
Unwanted pregnancy
Premature birth
Early separation
Step-parent

EFFECT OF NEGLECT IN CHILDHOOD
Behavioural disorders, e.g., conduct disorder
Externalizing—aggression, overactivity
Internalizing—anxiety, self-harm, suicidal ideation
Conduct disorder
Anxiety, e.g., PTSD
Depression
Eating disorders
Resilience

EXTREME EFFECT OF NEGLECT IN CHILDHOOD
Reduced brain size
Reduced brain activity

Reduced brain development
Deficit in processing facial emotion
Disinhibited attachment
Reduced emotional regulation

ADULT CONSEQUENCE OF CHILDHOOD NEGLECT
Drug dependence
Alcohol dependence
Anxiety
Depression
PTSD
Eating disorders
Obesity
Psychosis

DOMESTIC VIOLENCE
Twenty-five percent of all reported crimes
Ninety percent of children are in the same or an adjacent room where partner assault occurs at home
Areas of high unemployment
Economic deprivation
Personality disorder
Extreme jealousy

EFFECTS ON CHILD WITNESSES OF DOMESTIC VIOLENCE
Depends on developmental stage/gender/role

Disrupted sleep

Anxiety and other emotional disorders

Psychosomatic disorders

Conduct disorders

Inappropriate adult roles

Reduced school attendance/performance

Inappropriate coping skills, especially aggression

ASSESSMENT OF SUSPECTED ABUSE OR NEGLECT

Physician should have a high index of suspicion for abuse when evaluating an injured child, particularly with delayed seeking of medical care and inconsistent and frequently changing stories.

Obtain full history from multiple informants. Speak to them separately regarding events.

Information from child, parent, siblings, babysitter, school, primary care physician, and protective services may be indicated.

Children may be reluctant to disclose abuse.

Ask the child directly about means of discipline at home.

Ask the child directly about having been touched in private places or asked to do things to other people's privates.

Assess for inconsistency of reports.

Assessment of new onset of sleep disturbance, startled reaction, regression.

Decline in academic and social functioning and regression.

New psychiatric symptoms.

Assessment of attachment issues, failure to thrive, PTSD.

Behavioural difficulties.

Sexual acting out or sexually provocative behaviours.

PHYSICAL EXAMINATION OF SUSPECTED ABUSE OR NEGLECT

Multiple injuries at various stages of healing

History of failure to thrive

A history inconsistent with the injury

Bruises in the pattern of a belt or fingers

Spiral fracture or rib fractures

Burn in a cigarette shape

Head and eye injuries, hemorrhages on fundoscopic examination

Unexplained serious abdominal injuries

Any injuries to genitals

MANAGEMENT OF CHILD ABUSE AND NEGLECT

The following assessment can be followed if child abuse/neglect is identified:

- The initial goal of treatment is to ensure that the child is safe and to prevent further abuse
- This is typically done with the protective service agencies
- The child may be removed from the home and placed in a foster or group home or with one of his/her relatives who can act as legal guardian
- The abuser will require treatment, close monitoring, and support if the child is to remain in the home or return to the home at a later date
- Maintain child safety
- Physical treatment for child if indicated
- Ensure involvement of social services, school, and wider network

- Psychological intervention for child as indicated
- Parent-child interaction therapy
- Parenting programs that improve sensitivity of care and support parent
- Parent mental health treatment

PROTECTIVE FACTORS TO PREVENT CHILD MALTREATMENT

Child factors:
- Ability to recognize danger and adapt
- Ability to distance oneself from intense feelings
- Ability to imagine oneself at a time and place in the future in which the perpetrator is no longer present
- Good health
- Good school
- Adults outside the family who serve as positive role models/mentors
- Average or above average intelligence
- Hobbies or interest
- Good peer relationships and social skills
- Easy temperament
- Positive self-esteem
- Internal locus of control

Family factors:
- Secure attachment
- Parents working through of their own abuse history
- Supportive family environment

- Household rules and supervision
- Extended family support
- Family expectation of prosocial behaviour
- Middle to high socioeconomic status
- Access to healthcare and childcare
- Sufficient housing
- Steady parental employment
- Religious affiliation

CONCLUSION

Child maltreatment is defined as physical and emotional mistreatment, sexual abuse, neglect, child exploitation, and exposure to intimate partner violence. Child abuse has increased dramatically globally. It is likely due to an increase in awareness and reporting. Maltreatment is associated with significant developmental, psychological and physical impairment in childhood, adolescence and extending across the life span. All clinicians who come in contact with children should have a high index of suspicion for abuse potential when evaluating particularly non-accidentally injured children. Exploring risk factors and abuse circumstances could lead to early identification of a maltreated and abused child. Ensuring child safety must be the initial goal. Further management should be aimed at the child and caregiver. The assistance and support needed should be provided, including appropriate intervention for prevention and rehabilitation.

REFERENCES

Addo, A. S. (2013). Consultant child and adolescent psychiatry. Maltreatment: ASA UGMS. Glasgow, U.K.

Afifi, T. O. (2011). Child maltreatment in Canada: An understudied public health problem. *Canadian Journal of Public Health, 102*(6), 459–61.

Coghill, D., Graham, J., & Bonnar, S., et al. (2009). *Child and Adolescent Psychiatry.* Oxford, United Kingdom: Oxford University Press.

Public Health Agency of Canada. (2008). Canadian incidence study of reported child abuse and neglect—"Executive summary."

Stubbe, D. (2007). *Child and Adolescent Psychiatry.* Philadelphia, Pennsylvania, United States: Lippincott Williams & Wilkins.

Wikipedia.org. "Demographics of Canada."

World Health Organization. (2014). Health topics: "Child Maltreatment."

23. FAILURE TO THRIVE (FTT)

OBJECTIVES

This chapter will highlight the negative impact of failure to thrive (FTT) in children, as well as the identification, poverty correlations, early intervention, and prevention of FTT.

NEGATIVE IMPACT OF FAILURE TO THRIVE IN CHILDREN

Failure to thrive (FTT) serves as an early sign of children's vulnerability.

Although many children with FTT experience growth and cognitive recovery by school age, they continue to be at risk for poor growth and low academic achievement.

Early failure to thrive increases child's risk of having short stature, poor arithmetic performance, and poor work habits.

When FTT occurs in conjunction with additional threats to children's well being, such as neglect, the negative effects on children's behavioural, cognitive, and academic function are compounded.

IDENTIFICATION OF FAILURE TO THRIVE

Community studies indicate that up to 50% of children with FTT are not identified.

Growth screening to identify children with FTT and interdisciplinary interventions have been effective in promoting children's growth and development.

POVERTY CORRELATES WITH FTT

Poverty affects development regardless of growth interventions status.

In communities where there are social safeguards through public assistance programs, such as supplemental nutrition programs for women, infant, and children, and food stamp programs, the likelihood of severe FTT is reduced.

EARLY INTERVENTION

Early interventions targeted towards disadvantaged young children have much higher returns than later interventions.

Efforts to provide early intervention to vulnerable children and their families should be continued along with long-term-follow-up evaluations to assess and improve additional developmental risks.

HOME INTERVENTION

Home visiting attenuates some of the negative effects of early failure to thrive by promoting maternal sensitivity, enhancing mother-child relationship, and teaching the mother to respond to her child's need for interaction.

Beneficial effects include the mother becoming child-focused, and academic performance and work habits of the child improve.

PREVENTION OF FAILURE TO THRIVE

Growth screening to identify FTT and interdisciplinary intervention

Early home intervention mitigates many negative effects of FTT. It is effective in helping children to take advantage of academic opportunities.

Strategies are needed to protect children from the negative consequences of poverty through economic resources and opportunities for their families to provide responsive and stimulating caregiving environments.

CONCLUSION

Failure to thrive (FTT) continues to serve as an early sign of children's vulnerability. When FTT occurs, the negative effects on children's behavioural, cognitive, and academic function is compounded. Poverty is associated with FTT. Early intervention mitigates many negative effects of FTT.

REFERENCES

Black, M. M., Dubowitz, H., Krishnakumar, A., & Starr, Jr., R. H. (2007). Early intervention and recovery among children with failure to thrive: Follow-up at age 8. *Paediatrics, 120*(1), 59–69.

24. PEDIATRIC SOMATIZATION

OBJECTIVES

This chapter will discuss the epidemiology of somatization, somatization with co-occurring anxiety, negative impacts of somatization, and treatment of somatization, including family intervention.

EPIDEMIOLOGY OF SOMATIZATION

Somatic complaints are common among anxiety-disordered youth with more than 50% reporting at least one somatic complaint.

Somatic symptoms are equally common in children and youth with a principal diagnosis of separation anxiety, social anxiety, and generalized anxiety disorders (GAD).

Somatic complaints have been found to be more common among girls than boys in a community sample.

Somatic complaints among youth with anxiety disorders are usually not related to race or family income.

Children with anxiety disorders and somatic complaints have more severe anxiety and poorer global functioning.

SOMATIZATION WITH CO-OCCURRING ANXIETY

Somatic symptoms in youth with anxiety disorders may be associated with greater psychopathology.

Anxiety disorders occur in approximately 10% of youth and are associated with impairment in family, social, and academic functioning.

Untreated anxiety disorders run a chronic course and are "gateway" disorders associated with an increased risk for depression, substance-abuse problems, and educational underachievement.

NEGATIVE IMPACT OF SOMATIZATION

Children perform sub-optimally academically and are more likely to refuse school.

They often have co-occurring anxiety, mood, and substance-abuse problems, with poor family, social, and global functioning.

The severity of pre-treatment physical symptoms is associated with co-occurring mental health disorders.

Children presenting with a fabricated illness have potentially intermediate- to long-term adverse outcomes and are commonly referred for management to child protective services.

TREATMENT SOMATIZATION

Current research findings suggest that evaluation for anxiety disorder is warranted when children/youth present with frequent somatic complaints.

Treatment of anxiety with medication and CBT reduces somatic complaints.

Promoting awareness of physical symptoms of anxiety may facilitate improvement.

FAMILY INTERVENTION OF SOMATIZATION

Clinicians should actively avoid denying, minimizing, dismissing, challenging, or pushing away any of the concerns expressed by the family.

Rather, use ongoing contact to build a solid therapeutic alliance and provide support with regard to family concern and task.

Instead of giving primary attention to the symptoms, choose interventions that simultaneously facilitate engagement for understanding of family functioning and encourage a focus on active problem-solving task.

Collaboration with the therapeutic team and family will share responsibility for trying to understand the problem and finding a solution for demanding further tests.

CONCLUSION

Somatic complaints are common among anxiety disordered children and youth. Clinicians should actively avoid minimizing and dismissing any of the concerns expressed by the family. Collaboration with the therapeutic team and family is critical in investigating the issue and uncovering a solution.

REFERENCES

Crawley, S. A., et al. (2014). Somatic Complaints in Anxious Youth. *Hum Dev, 45*(4), 398–407.

Kendall, P. C., Crawley, S. A., et al. (2014). Somatic complaints in anxious youth. *Child Psychiatry Hum Dev., 45*(4), 398–407/s.

Kozlowska, K. Foley, S., & Savage, B. (2012). Fabricated illness: Working within the family system to find a pathway to health. *Family Process, 51*(4), 570–587.

25. LEARNING DISORDERS

OBJECTIVES
Learning disorders and co-occurring disorders will be identified. Assessment of types of disabilities for specialized service requirements, care plan, residential service and community participation will be discussed.

INTRODUCTION
People with learning disabilities are susceptible to mental illness. This disorder is uncommon in adult psychiatric services. Learning disorders are often associated with developmental delay, Tourette's syndrome, ASD, ADHD, and epilepsy-related disorders. If the above conditions are established before adulthood, they are often associated with educational problems, even if intellect is unimpaired.

INTELLECTUAL DEVELOPMENTAL DISORDER
Refers to sub-average general intellectual functioning in terms of cognitive functioning concurrently with communication, home living, social/interpersonal skills, use of community resources, self-direction, functional academic skills, leisure, and health and safety.

GLOBAL DEVELOPMENTAL DELAY

This diagnosis is reserved for children under the age of 5 years who fail to meet expected developmental milestones in several areas of intellectual functioning, and severity level cannot be assessed as they are too young to participate in standardized testing. They require reassessment after a period of time.

DUAL DIAGNOSIS

The phrase "dual diagnosis" was introduced in the USA (1988) to draw attention to the needs of people with mental retardation who have mental illness.

Recently confusion has arisen because of the use of the same term to describe people with mental illness who misuse substances.

ASSESSMENT

There should be a diagnostic assessment of the child's level of learning disability.

The cause of the intellectual impairment, identification of any other developmental disorders, and identification of acquired mental and physical disorders should be diagnosed.

Emotional and behavioural consequences of illness should be identified.

Risk assessment should consider, from others, the child's vulnerability to harm and severe self-neglect.

There should be an assessment of child/adolescent's decision-making capacity.

These assessments should lead to the construction of a care plan.

TYPES OF DISABILITIES

Secondary and tertiary disabilities are the impaired performances that are not directly attributable to intellectual impairment or mental illness but follow from frequent consequences, such as unemployment.

Common social consequences of learning disorders and severe mental illness include dependency on a caregiver, unemployment, poverty, and lack of relationships.

Psychological consequences include low self-esteem, lack of identity, loneliness, and boredom.

Tertiary disability: A person who repeatedly experiences demands that they cannot meet due to their impairment will learn methods that result in avoidance behaviour.

Comorbidity, such as ASD, ADHD, and epilepsy, is often a problem.

SERVICE MODEL

Effective models of rehabilitation for people with a learning disability and severe enduring mental illness require recognition.

These children need support for personal development.

They need treatment of episode of illness, prevention of recurrence, and rehabilitation because of their illness.

SPECIALIZED SERVICE REQUIREMENTS AND CARE PLAN

Health: physical and mental

Emotional well-being

Quality of life

Protection: the person with mild impairment may live with their caregivers. Those who have a severe disability with multiple co-occurring disorders may have to be placed in residential care.

Person's wishes and decision-making capacity need to be supported by advocacy and legal protection.

Consultation needs to be carried out with people, such as family, with an interest in the patient's welfare.

RESIDENTIAL SERVICE

Setting: environmental and social requirements (e.g., space, garden, noise, traffic, neighbours)

Building: special adaptation or constraints required for access, privacy or safety, ramps, gates or stairs/all one level, safety glass, sensor to alert staff

Domestic equipment: Any special arrangements for toilet, bath/shower, etc.

Staffing level: Day and night with explanation of reasons for specified minimum level of staffing

Staff characteristics: Special skills or other characteristics required, including qualifications, gender, build, responsiveness to specific client characteristics

Client numbers: Maximum and minimum number of residents the person can live with and an explanation for these specifications

Client mix: issues that affect compatibility

Risk management: Any special arrangements required to respond to risk assessment, including legal protection, procedure, skills, supervision arrangement, etc.

Other factors: Such as contact with family, continuity of other relationships, transport, or anything specifically needed to promote service aims

Day activities: Same list of considerations adopted for activities, such as employment and vocational activities

Education and training: Social, recreational, and leisure activities

Therapeutic activities

Visiting services: Determined by individual assessment

COMMUNITY PARTICIPATION

Community integration interventions appear to be effective in enhancing the inclusion of children and adolescents with neurodevelopmental and intellectual disabilities. There is a need for the development of programs to facilitate friendships alongside recreational participation, including typically developing peers, and accommodating individual impairments. Community integration facilitates friendship development and improves self-esteem and quality of life.

CONCLUSION

Children with learning disabilities are susceptible to mental illness. Learning disorders are often associated with developmental delay, as well as Tourette's syndrome, ASD, ADHD, and epilepsy-related disorders. There should be a diagnostic assessment to identify any other developmental, mental, and physical disorders. Effective models of rehabilitation for children with a learning disability and a severe enduring mental illness require recognition and need support for personal development, treatment of illness, and rehabilitation of their disabilities.

REFERENCES

Andrews, J., et al. (2015). Community participation interventions for children and adolescents with a neurodevelopmental intellectual disability: a systemic review. *Disabil Rehabil,* *37*(10), 825–833.

Holloway, F., Kalidindi, S., Killaspy, H. & Roberts, G. (eds.). (2015). *Enabling Recovery: The Principles and Practice of Rehabilitation Psychiatry* (2nd ed.). London, UK: RCPsych Publications.

University of Toronto. (1998). MCCQE Review notes and Lecture series. Toronto, Canada: Faculty of Medicine, University of Toronto.

26. JUVENILE SUBSTANCE ABUSE

OBJECTIVES

This chapter will discuss the global epidemiology and risk factors for developing substance-abuse disorder. Protective factors, stages of developing abuse, psychiatric comorbidities, screening, assessment, multimodal treatment, and prevention will also be covered.

INTRODUCTION

Rates of illicit drug abuse during the last 30 years have risen dramatically. A large proportion of the disease burden and deaths of young people in developed nations is attributable to the misuse of alcohol and drugs. In general substance abuse is a disorder that starts in adolescence or early adulthood. It complicates with other psychiatric comorbidities and often has serious negative consequences.

EPIDEMIOLOGY

It is estimated that in the US over 5 million teenagers meet the diagnostic criteria for a substance-abuse disorder. It is the second most commonly diagnosed psychiatric disorder in youth, at an estimated 12.2% by age 16.

FINDINGS FROM THE STUDENT DRUG USE SURVEY 2009, ONTARIO, CANADA

Past year of drug use in a total sample of 9,112 student in grades 7–12:

(Q: Have you used this substance at least once in the past year?)

Alcohol: 58.2%

Cannabis: 25.6%

Binge drinking in the past 4 weeks (5+ drinks): 24.7%

Non-medicinal opioids: 17.8%

Tobacco: 11.7%

Ecstasy: 3.2%

Cocaine: 2.6%

LSD: 1.8%

Heroin: 0.7%

Crystal meth: 0.5%

Groups not included in this data include street youth, youth on aboriginal reserves, youth residing in correctional facilities—all these groups have higher rates of use.

According to UNICEF, street children younger than 18 years of age are estimated to number at around 10 million to 100 million worldwide, mostly living in developing countries.

Substance abuse, mental and physical health problems among street children are serious issues.

Baer et al. (2003) found that 69% of their homeless sample met the criteria for dependence on at least one substance.

Soyibo and Lee (1997) found that among Jamaican school-attending adolescents rates of alcohol were 50.2%, tobacco 16.6%, marijuana 10.2%, cocaine 2.2%, and heroin use of 1.13%, respectively.

A survey of 17,215 students aged 12–20 years from Panama, Costa Rica, and Guatemala conducted in 2000–2001 showed lifetime substance-abuse rates of alcohol abuse 61.6%, cigarette use 40.4%, marijuana use 6.2%, and other drug use 18.3% (Dormitzer et al., 2004).

A survey of 1,296 students from 17 schools in Nairobi, Kenya, with a mean age of 17 years, showed substance-abuse rates of alcohol 9.3%, cigarettes 5.3%; use was more common and began as early as before the age of 11 (Ndetei et al., 2009).

A survey of 1,720 Turkish university students with a mean age of 21.5 years reported lifetime use of cannabis 5.9%, ecstasy 1.7%, heroin 0.2%, and cocaine 0.4% (Ilhan et al., 2006).

A study among undergraduate medical students in two medical colleges in Calcutta, India, indicated a prevalence of total and current drug abusers of 48.9% and 27.9% respectively. Commonly used drugs included alcohol and tobacco (Naskar & Bhattacharya, 1999).

A survey of 1,118 adolescents between Grades 8–9 in an urban area of Cape Town, South Africa were examined. Results indicated adolescents first tried either alcohol or cigarettes, followed by cannabis and then inhalants (Morojele et al., 2011).

RISK FACTORS FOR DEVELOPING SUBSTANCE-ABUSE PROBLEMS

Chaotic home environment

Parental substance abuse

Parental mental illness

Ineffective parenting

Lack of parental involvement

Perceived parental/peer/community approval of drug use

Poor social coping skills
History of abuse
Early use of substances
Peers who use substances
Associating with conduct disorder peers
Concurrent depression/anxiety/conduct disorder
Chronic medical condition
Failing school/poor school performance
Learning disability
Gay/lesbian youth

PROTECTIVE FACTORS

Personal belief in God: Studies suggest that religious adolescents engage in less deviant behaviour.

Parental religiosity: Parents communicate values regarding the behaviour of their children and likely support and monitor their adolescents' behaviour.

Positive family interaction patterns: Cohesive families communicate better and provide support to adolescents.

Positive student-teacher interaction: a tremendous source of support when adolescents lack support from parents.

Positive adjustment during adolescence.

STAGES OF SUBSTANCE USE

Curiosity → Experimentation → Regular use → Harmful use → Dependence

Terminology

Substance use: At least once in the past year

Substance misuse: Emergence of a pattern of use

Substance abuse: Adverse consequences related to the use of a substance; use in situations that are hazardous.

Substance dependence: Regular use with associated impairment, inability to control use, use despite consequences, physiological symptoms, tolerance and withdrawal tolerance; need to increase the amount to achieve the desired effect or diminished effect with continued use of the same amount.

Withdrawal of psychoactive substance: Specific syndromes following cessation of regular use; withdrawal effects when substance discontinued or the same or a related substance is taken to relieve or avoid withdrawal symptoms.

Intoxication: Maladaptive behaviour associated with recent drug ingestion. The effects of intoxication of any drug can vary widely among persons and depend on such factors as dose, circumstances, and underlying personality.

Addiction: a nonspecific lay term which implies psychological dependency, drug-seeking behaviour, physical dependence and tolerance, and associated deterioration of physical and mental health.

PATHWAYS OF JUVENILE SUBSTANCE ABUSE

Experimenting with alcohol and illicit drugs is fairly common among adolescents. Young people cite many reasons for such behaviour, including peer pressure, curiosity, fun and availability. They may also use alcohol and drugs to deal with problems or negative feelings.

DYNAMIC ISSUES

Self-medication: Amelioration of specific symptoms

Use of marijuana for ADHD

Use of alcohol for anxiety

To blunt intolerable affect states of emotional, physical, sexual abuse

JUVENILE SUBSTANCE ABUSE AND PSYCHIATRIC COMORBIDITIES

Studies suggest about 60% of adolescents with substance-abuse problems also have one or more co-occurring disorders. The most common of these are:

A) Oppositional Defiant Disorder: Up to 80% of substance-abuse adolescents meet the diagnostic criteria for ODD. Many symptoms contained within the disorder are related to substance abuse. ODD patients have a trend of experiencing higher rates of adolescent-onset substance abuse.

B) Conduct Disorder: CD is the biggest risk factor associated with childhood psychopathologic disorder (leading to substance abuse 80% to 90% of the time). Substance abuse may accelerate the emergence of conduct disorder. Additive risk factors when comorbid with other disorders, e.g., ADHD, depression, bipolar, and anxiety disorder.

C) ADHD: Psychiatric comorbidity (e.g., ODD, CD, anxiety, depression), school failure, poor peer relationships, legal difficulties, accidents and injuries, family conflicts, parent stress, and alcohol and illicit drug abuse.

Does the pharmacotherapy of ADHD give rise to later substance abuse?

A meta-analytic review of the literature examining the impact of early medication treatment for ADHD in childhood on subsequent substance-abuse disorder outcomes in adolescent and young adult years shows that stimulant pharmacotherapy for ADHD significantly decreases the risk for subsequent substance-use disorder.

D) Anxiety Disorders: 20% to 30% of adolescents with substance abuse have social anxiety disorder; 40% of high school seniors report using drugs to "reduce anxiety."

E) Depression: 30% to 40% substance abuse with depression; 40% to 50% substance abuse with dysthymia; 10% to 20% substance abuse with dysthymia + depression

F) Bipolar Disorder: Assess all adolescents with binge substance abuse for bipolar disorder and bipolar disorder for substance abuse

G) Psychotic Disorder: Most frequently psychosis occurs as a consequence of illicit drug use

CONSIDER SCREENING FOR SUBSTANCE ABUSE

Sudden drop in academics and increased school disciplinary action

Recent unexplained loss of interest in sports/pastimes

Rapid changes of mood: low mood, irritability, anger

Onset of antisocial behaviour, association with substance abuser

Early drinking (under 15 years old)

C-R-A-F-F-T SUBSTANCE ABUSE SCREENING QUESTIONNAIRES

Ever ridden in a CAR while high on drugs or alcohol?

Ever use drugs or alcohol to RELAX?

Ever use drugs or alcohol while ALONE?

Does FAMILY or FRIEND criticize about drinking/drug use?

Ever gotten into TROUBLE while using alcohol/drugs?

ASSESSMENT FOR SUBSTANCE ABUSE

Historic data should be collected from multiple sources.

Patient alone likely to minimize or deny use.

Determine if youth has drug use, abuse, or dependence.

Try to determine how many substances are being used and how available they are.

Assess family and home situation, level of communication, parental supervision and support.

Obtain a family history of substance abuse/mental illness.

Assess for other psychiatric comorbidities.

A comprehensive physical examination, blood count, liver function tests, toxicology (drug) screen.

MULTIMODAL TREATMENT OF SUBSTANCE USE DISORDERS

Psychoeducation of parents and youth about the nature of the illness.

Family therapy is critical for treatment of improving parent/child communication, lack of parental involvement, and need for clear family rules.

Set up a plan to avoid situations that trigger substance abuse, e.g., friends or hangouts.

Cognitive behavioural therapy may be used to target thinking errors and to increase self-control.

Group therapy may be helpful; possible risk of younger and more naive members learning "bad habits" from other group members.

School interventions may be required to motivate and engage child in academic success.

Substance-abuse counselling in a school setting is often beneficial.

Inpatient rehabilitation may be required for drug dependence.

Medication management aimed at treating intoxication states and withdrawal conditions, preventing continued use, and providing narcotic maintenance.

PSYCHOPHARMACOLOGICAL STRATEGIES

Medication is part of a multimodal treatment plan to:

- Reduce urge or craving
- Treat underlying comorbidity, e.g., ADHD, ODD, CD, bipolar disorder, depression, anxiety
- Preventive therapy: treating risk factors, i.e., psychopathology
- Avoid the potential for misuse, drug interaction

PREVENTION

Parents, especially mothers, should be targeted in the campaign against drug use so that they are made aware of the risks that their children are exposed to while in school and educated on how to deal with the use of drugs.

Mothers are more emotionally attached to their children and are more likely than fathers to spend quality time with their children.

Aggressive psychoeducation to parent and child regarding substance abuse; positive and open communication to be maintained between parents and child.

Discussion of known risk factors (e.g., CD); close monitoring in high-risk cases (e.g., urine toxicology).

Education on the dangers of drug use should begin early, while students are still in primary school and before they attain the age of 11 years. Education should be offered continuously across all age groups.

Aggressive approaches should be adopted in the fight against drug use with schools forming linkages with the parents.

Regulatory interventions aiming to increase price, reduce availability and accessibility of substances, restrict settings of use, and raise legal purchase age are effective in reducing the use of alcohol and tobacco and related harms.

CONCLUSION

Epidemiological studies indicate that the prevalence of juvenile substance abuse is rising and is among the most prevalent psychiatric disorders in young people. It is often associated with comorbid psychopathology. Treatment of substance abuse is multimodal, and family is central with open communication at home. Psychotherapy combined with pharmacotherapy can be effective in youth with substance-abuse problems. Aggressive treatment of comorbid psychopathology may reduce ultimate substance-abuse disorders. Educating and improving awareness among youth and parents are key factors for the prevention of substance-abuse disorders.

REFERENCES

American Psychiatric Association. (2013). Diagnostic and statistical manual of mental disorders (5th ed.). Arlington, VA, US: American Psychiatric Publishing, Inc.

Baer, J., Ginzler, J. A. & Peterson, P. L. (2003). DSM-IV alcohol and substance abuse and dependence in homeless youth. *Journal of Studies on Alcohol.*

Blum, R. et al. (2003). Adolescent health in the Caribbean: Risk & protective factors. *American Journal of Public Health,* 93(1), 456–460.

Bukstein, O. et al. (2005). Practice parameter for the assessment & treatment of children & adolescents with substance abuse disorders. *J Am Acad Adol Psych,* 44(6), 609–621.

Georgiades, K. & Boyle, M. H. (2007). Adolescent tobacco and cannabis use: young adult outcomes from the Ontario Child Health Study. *J Child Psychol Psychiatry,* 48(7), 724–731.

Hotton, T. et al. (2004). Alcohol And drug use in early adolescence. *Health Reports,* 15(3), Statistics Canada, Catalogue No. 82-003.

Ilhan, I. et al. (2009). Prevalence & sociodemographic correlates of substance abuse in a university-student sample in turkey. *Int J Public health,* 54, 40–44.

Knight, J. R. et al. (2003). Validity of the CRAFFT substance abuse screening test among adolescent clinic patients. *Arch Pediat Adolesc Med,* 156, 607–614.

Morojele, N., Myers, B., Townsend, L., Lombard, C., Plüddemann, A., Carney, T., Petersen Williams, P., Padayachee, T., Nel, E. & Nkosi, S. (2013). Survey on Substance Use, Risk Behaviour and Mental Health among Grade 8–10 Learners in Western Cape Provincial Schools, 2011. Cape Town: South African Medical Research Council.

Naskar, N.N. & Bhattacharya, S.K. (1999). A study on drug abuse among the undergraduate medical students in Calcutta. *J Indian Med Assoc., 97*(1), 20–21.

Ndetei, D. et al. (2009). Patterns of Drug abuse in public secondary schools in Kenya. *Substance Abuse, 30,* 69–78.

Patrick, M. E., Collins, L. M., Smith, E., Caldwell, L., Flisher, A., & Wegner, L. (2009). A prospective longitudinal model of substance use onset among South African adolescents. *Subst Use Misuse, 44*(5), 647–662.

Souza, R. & deLeon, M. (2007). Reducing harm caused by substance use in adolescents. The Lancet, 369, 2157–2158.

Soyibo, K. & Lee, M. G. (1997). Use of alcohol, tobacco and non-prescription drugs among Jamaican high school students. *West Indian Med J., 46,* 111–114.

Stubbe, D. (2007). *Child and Adolescent Psychiatry.* Philadelphia, Pennsylvania, United States: Lippincott Williams & Wilkins.

Wilens, T. (1996). Adolescent Substance abuse: focus on psychiatric comorbidity. Clinical research program in Paediatric psychopharmacology.

27. INTERNET, VIDEO GAMING, AND GAMBLING ADDICTION IN ADOLESCENTS

OBJECTIVES

This chapter will explain possible causes of excessive internet use, video gaming and gambling, as well as the diagnostic criteria, risk factors, negative impact, comorbidity, and treatment for these addictions.

INTRODUCTION

Internet use and video-game play are widespread forms of entertainment and have become an ever-increasing part of children and adolescents' lives. Gambling is problematic as well.

Video-game playing has become a very popular activity among adolescents.

Its impact on the mental health and well-being of players is just beginning to be explored.

It is not clear whether problematic internet use is associated with other risky behaviours such as substance use.

Murad Bakht, FRCP (C)

INTERNET ADDICTION

Why does excessive internet use occur?

Individuals with psychosocial problems (e.g., depression and loneliness) have negative perceptions of their social competence.

Such individuals prefer computer-mediated interactions to face-to-face interactions, as the former is perceived to be less threatening.

Individuals also perceive themselves as being more efficient in an online setting.

This preference leads to excessive and compulsive use of computer-mediated interactions, which then creates problems at school and at home.

Diagnostic criteria for identifying internet addiction

The following diagnostic criteria are based on the work of Beard and Wolf (2001). All of the following must be present:

- Is preoccupied and has stayed online with the internet longer than originally intended
- Needs to use the internet with increased amounts of time in order to achieve satisfaction
- Has made unsuccessful efforts to control, cut back, or stop internet use
- Is restless, moody, depressed, or irritable when attempting to cut down or stop internet use

And at least one of the following:

- Has jeopardized or risked the loss of a significant relationship or educational opportunity because of the internet

- Has lied to family members, therapist, or others to conceal the extent of involvement with the internet
- Uses the internet as a way of escaping from problems or relieving a dysphoric mood, e.g., feeling of helplessness, guilt, anxiety, or depression

Risk factor for problematic internet use

Lack of social activity

Anxiety symptoms

Problematic tobacco and alcohol consumption

Video game addiction

Poor relationship with family

Negative impact of internet addiction

Social impairment

Vocational impairment

Financial impairment

Legal problems

Internet addiction, and comorbidity

Substance abuse, mood, anxiety, and psychotic disorders

Compulsive buying, gambling, pyromania, and compulsive sexual behaviour

Physical and sexual abuse in childhood

Borderline, narcissistic, and antisocial personality disorder

Treatment for internet addiction

Cognitive behavioural therapy (CBT)

Treat comorbid psychiatric disorders

Problem-solving supportive therapy

Changing to a healthy lifestyle

VIDEO-GAME ADDICTION

Reasons why males play video games more than females

The content of the game: Most video games have traditionally masculine images.

Socialization: Women are not encouraged to express aggression in public and feel uncomfortable with games of combat or war.

Sex differences: Males on average have better visual and spatial skills, particularly depth perception, which is essential for good game playing. Therefore, male players score higher than females and persist in playing.

Diagnostic criteria for video-game addiction

Salience: This occurs when video game play becomes the most important activity in a person's life, dominating their thinking (cognitive distortion), feelings, cravings, and behaviour (deterioration of socialized behaviour)

Mood modification: Subjective experience as a consequence of playing and seen as a coping strategy, e.g., experience of arousing a "buzz" or a "high"

Or paradoxically, a tranquillizing feeling of "escape"

Or numbing tolerance: this is the process whereby increased amounts of video game play are required to achieve the mood modifying effects

Withdrawal symptoms: unpleasant feeling state/or physical effects that occur when video game play is discontinued or suddenly reduced (shakes, moodiness, irritability)

Conflict: interpersonal conflicts with family, school, work, social life, hobbies, and interests

Subjective feeling of loss of control spending too much time engaged in video game play

Relapse: tendency for repeated reversions to earlier patterns of video-game play after periods of abstinence or control

Medical complication of video-game addiction

Risk of epileptic seizure

Obesity

Blisters, calluses, sore tendons, and numbness of fingers, hands, and elbows

Wrist pain, neck pain, elbow pain, tenosynovitis

Hallucinations, enuresis, encopresis

Social impact of video-game addiction

Excessive video game playing may prevent children and adolescents from participating in educational and sporting activities

Poor social skills

Social isolation and anxiety

Treatment for video-game addiction

Cognitive behavioural modification therapy

Family therapy

Changing to a healthy lifestyle

Treat psychiatric and medical comorbidity

Murad Bakht, FRCP (C)

GAMBLING ADDICTION

Introduction

Excessive gambling is no different from alcohol and illicit drug addiction in terms of the core components of addiction.

Epidemiology of gambling

Internationally, adolescent gambling is increasingly recognized as an important mental and public health issue.

Adolescent problem gambling has reported prevalence rates ranging from 2% to 7.4%.

A survey in Ontario, Canada, in 2000, found that 7.5% of students in grades 7–13 met the criteria for at-risk gambling and 5.8% met the criteria for problem gambling.

A national survey of 12- to 18-year-olds from Finland found 44% had gambled during the past 6 months.

Etiological factors of gambling

Loss of parent

Inappropriate parental discipline

Exposure to/availability of gambling activities for adolescents

A family emphasis on material and financial support

Increased stress and inability to cope with negative life events increase severity of gambling

Risk factors for gambling addiction

Low self-esteem

Depressive mood

Victim of physical or sexual abuse

Poor school performance
History of delinquency (poor impulse control)
Being male
Parental history of addiction and parenting styles
Family and community facilitate gambling venues
Lack of connection to the school community
Learning disorders
Disinhibition, boredom, lack of self-discipline
Negative life events

Gambling and comorbidity
Adolescent gamblers are more likely to:
- Smoke tobacco
- Drink alcohol
- Smoke illicit drugs
- Have experienced negative life events

Pathological gambling and comorbidity
Mood disorders, especially depression
Anxiety disorders, including panic disorder and OCD
Learning disorders and ADHD
Alcohol and other substance use

DSM-5 CRITERIA FOR GAMBLING DISORDERS
Recurrent, problematic for at least four of the following gambling behaviours with significant impairment or distress in a 12-month period:

- Needs to gamble with increasing amounts of money to achieve desired excitement
- Is restless or irritable when attempting to stop or cut down gambling
- Unsuccessful attempt(s) to cut down or stop gambling
- Often preoccupied with thoughts of gambling
- Often gambles when feeling distressed
- After losing money often returns another day hoping to win
- Lies to conceal the extent of involvement in gambling
- Has jeopardized or lost a significant relationship, job, or educational opportunity
- Relies on others to provide money to relieve desperate financial situation caused by gambling

Prevention of underage problem gambling

Prevention efforts are directed towards non-users (primary prevention), screening for potential problems (secondary prevention), and treatment (tertiary prevention)

Fundamental in a successful prevention program is to educate children in primary school since they have not yet started engaging in gambling behaviour

Harm reduction and abstinence would be a secondary prevention strategy

Tertiary prevention strategies are designed as harm minimization for individuals who cannot be prevented from engaging in particularly risky behaviours

Adolescents with gambling problems, in general, tend not to present themselves for treatment

Treatment for gambling addiction

Fear of being identified and stigma are often reasons attributed to failure to seek treatment

Legal difficulties, family pressure, or other psychiatric condition(s) brings the gambler into treatment

Gamblers Anonymous (GA) is the most effective treatment with inspirational group therapy

Hospitalization by removal from environment to decrease craving

Treat comorbid condition

Insight-oriented psychotherapy may help

The McGill treatment paradigm

Initial process:
- Establishing mutual trust and respect
- Assessment and setting of individual goals
- Assessment of readiness to change

Goals of therapy:
- Understanding the motivations for gambling
- Analysis of gambling episodes: Triggers → Emotional reactions and rationalizations → Behaviour → Consequences
- Establishing a baseline of gambling behaviour and encouraging a decrease in gambling
- Challenging cognitive distortions
- Establishing the underlying causes of stress and anxiety
- Evaluating and improving coping abilities
- Rebuilding healthy interpersonal relationships

- Restructuring free time
- Fostering effective money-management skills
- Relapse prevention

CONCLUSION

Internet use and video-game playing by children and adolescents have become popular activities. Their impact on the mental health and well-being of players is just beginning to be explored. To identify the medical and psychosocial impact of video-game addiction and excessive internet use, proper diagnosis is needed so that appropriate treatment can be provided. In addition, excessive gambling is no different from alcohol and illicit drug addiction in terms of core components of addiction. Diagnosis highlights the severity and comorbidity. Treatment of problem gambling and prevention needs to be ensured.

REFERENCES

American Psychiatric Association. (2013). Diagnostic and statistical manual of mental disorders (5th ed.). Arlington, VA, US: American Psychiatric Publishing, Inc.

Essau, C. A. & Delfabbro, R. (Eds.) (2008). *Adolescent Addiction: Epidemiology, Assessment, and Treatment (Practical Resources for the Mental Health Professional)* (1st ed.). New York: Elsevier Inc.

28. CYBERBULLYING

OBJECTIVES

This chapter will define cyberbullying, explain how cyberbullies operate, and identify types of cyberbullying, as well as the effects of cyberbullying on the victim and adult outcomes of childhood bullying. Factors co-occurring with cyberbullying and suicide, the correlation of cyberbullying and suicide, impact at school, reasons cited by students for not reporting to school, warning signs of victims affected by cyberbullying, interventions, parents' role, and school support will be covered. Finally, online safety, solutions, and recourses will be discussed.

SOCIAL MEDIA

Using social media websites is among the most common activities of today's children and adolescents.

Any website that allows social interaction is considered a social media site.

Such sites offer today's youth a portal for entertainment and communication and have grown rapidly in recent years.

SOCIAL MEDIA SITES

Social networking sites, such as Facebook, Twitter, Instagram, Snapchat

Gaming sites and virtual worlds, such as Club Penguin, Second Life, Sims, Roblox

Video sites, such as YouTube, Vine, Netflix, blogs, or vlogs (video blogs)

ROLE OF FRONTLINE CLINICIANS

It is important that parents become aware of the nature of social media sites.

Not all of them are healthy environments for children and adolescents.

Frontline clinicians, such as family physicians, pediatricians, and mental health clinicians are in a unique position to help families understand these sites, encourage healthy use, and urge parents to monitor for potential problems with cyberbullying.

WHAT IS CYBERBULLYING?

Definition: The use of electronic communication to bully a person, typically by sending messages of an intimidating or threatening nature.

Girls: Spreading rumours, secrets, posting and sending messages and pictures that make fun of or exclude people.

Boys: Messages tend to be of a sexual nature and may include threats to fight or hurts others.

HOW CYBERBULLIES OPERATE

Sending mean, vulgar, or threatening messages or images

Posting sensitive, private information about another person

Pretending to be someone else in order to make that person look bad

Intentionally excluding someone from an online group

Using the internet, smartphone, anonymous blogs, and social media to harass, intimidate, threaten or retaliate against enemies by spreading rumours

Posting inappropriate or unflattering pictures and excluding others

Many teens are harassed when someone steals their password or other personal information and sends damaging messages from their e-mail, personal website, or social networking pages.

A NEW FACE FOR AN OLD MONSTER

Bullying has been around for generations

Cyberbullying is the 21st-century version

Direct bullying: physical contact including hitting, punching and shoving, usually in a contained location (playground, locker room)

Limited audience; responsible party easily identified

Cyberbullying: emotional abuse can occur at any time and any place

Victims can run, but nowhere to hide

Large audience

Bully may be anonymous or at the very least veiled by the protection provided by the computer screen

TYPES OF CYBERBULLYING

Direct: sent to victim directly; intimidating, threatening, malicious messages

Twitter, Facebook, text messages, apps, blogs, instant messages, chatroom groups ganging up on one person

Willful and often repeated

By proxy: posing to be the victim after hacking into account or setting up a fake account in victim's name

Bully sends cruel, hateful messages

Sometimes gets others involved (sends rumour to an anonymous blog to post)

Victim gets blamed for attacks, punished by parents, loses friends

EFFECTS

Knowing the cyberbully can make the attack feel more personal

An anonymous attack can make the victim feel more vulnerable

Because there are so many possible avenues to inflict the attack, some victims report feeling like there is no escape from cyberbullying.

Depression with suicidal ideation

Anxiety, poor self-esteem

Psychosomatic symptoms, including headaches, difficulty sleeping

Intensified feelings of humiliation and isolation

Some victims found cyberbullying more devastating than direct bullying.

ADULT OUTCOMES OF CHILDHOOD BULLYING

Children who are frequently bullied continued to be at risk for a wide range of poor social, health, and economic outcomes in adult life.

FACTORS CO-OCCURRING WITH CYBERBULLYING AND SUICIDE

Depression

Social withdrawal

Disability

Social helplessness or other psychiatric morbidity

IMPACT AT SCHOOL

Although most cyberbullying occurs outside of school, it often begins with incidents that occurred during school.

Impact at school is evident:

- Desire to avoid school
- Lower grades
- Difficulty concentrating
- Feeling unsafe throughout the school day

CORRELATION BETWEEN CYBERBULLYING AND SUICIDE

Bullied youth—both the offender and target—were more likely to report suicidal thoughts and to have previously attempted suicide.

Being a target of bullying significantly increases the risk of suicide ideation in pre-adolescent children.

Cyberbullying victims were 1.9 times more likely to have attempted suicide.

Cyberbullying offenders were 1.5 times more likely to have attempted suicide.

Most victims of cyberbullying do not commit suicide.

Those who do usually have experienced a host of other issues, making it difficult to isolate the effect of cyberbullying.

Even one death due to cyberbullying is too many.

There is a relationship between bullying and suicide, however, no conclusive statistical evidence has shown that a cyberbullying incident directly leads to or causes suicide.

While by itself it is unlikely to lead to suicide, it may aggravate the victim's existing vulnerabilities.

It exacerbates instability and hopelessness in the minds of adolescents already struggling with stressful life circumstances.

Victims of cyberbullying reported more suicidal ideation than those who experienced physical or verbal bullying.

Suicide in youth arises from a complex interplay of various biological, psychological, and social factors of which bullying may be one factor.

VICTIMS

Victims often are unwilling to come forward.

They may tell friends, but most do not alert adults.

Research shows no relationship between help-seeking and cyberbullying, even though such a relationship exists with traditional bullying.

This may be explained by:

- Fear of losing access to their technology if they tell adults
- Fear the cyberbully will retaliate further
- Fear adults cannot do anything to stop it even if they tried or will make the situation worse
- Fear they will not be believed, or they will be blamed for their own aggressive response to the cyberbullying
- Fear the situation will be trivialized

REASONS CITED BY STUDENTS FOR NOT REPORTING CYBERBULLYING TO SCHOOL

They do not know who is doing it.

They lack confidence in educators' ability to understand or address the situation appropriately.

If it is occurring outside school, it is not clear to them why they should tell school personnel.

They are embarrassed.

They worry about being labelled "a rat" or "snitch."

WARNING SIGNS

Skipping activities that they used to enjoy

Spending more time alone in their rooms

Lack of eating or sleeping

Declining grades

Withdrawal from family and friends or reluctance to attend school and social events

Making negative statements about themselves and engaging in negative self-talk

Avoiding conversations and spending an unusual amount of time on the computer or cell phone

Quickly switching screens or closing programs when parent/guardian walks by the computer

STATISTICS

Nearly 43% of kids have been bullied online.

One in four has had it happen more than once.

Seventy percent of students report seeing frequent bullying online.

Over 80% of teens use a cellphone regularly, making it the most common medium for cyberbullying.

Eighty-one percent of young people think bullying online is easier to get away with than bullying in person.

Ninety percent of teens who have seen social-media bullying say they have ignored it.

Only 1 in 10 victims will inform a parent or trusted adult of their abuse.

Girls are about twice as likely as boys to be victims and perpetrators of cyberbullying.

Comments include: "go kill your self," "why aren't you dead?" "nobody likes you."

INTERVENTIONS

Block the sender

Ignore the message

Alert someone

Report the bully

Ask the bully to stop

Keep evidence of cyberbullying—though this can be emotionally damaging to the victim because it is not easily forgotten

Get the authorities to track down the ISP number

Contact the ISP

Report abuse in message board

Change email address

Don't visit certain sites

ADDITIONAL INTERVENTIONS

Focus on EMPOWERING students in terms of digital literacy to improve:
- Technological skills
- Critical thinking and problem-solving skills

- E-safety and assessing their own online risks
- Knowledge about cyberbullying and its effects
- Most students do not know how to keep themselves safe in cyberspace

Rather than trying to remove all risk (which is difficult to do), it is better to help students cope by strategizing with them on how to avoid negative situations.

ROLE OF FRONTLINE CLINICIANS

Frontline clinicians, such as family physicians, pediatricians, and mental-health clinicians should educate themselves on the warning signs of bullying, its effects, and interventions.

They are in a unique position to help families understand these websites and to help parents.

They should inform parents and children about the risks and consequences and include questions on bullying as part of initial and follow-up visits.

RISK ASSESSMENT OF BULLYING VICTIM

Ask about specific behaviours, not just if they have been bullied.

Detailed history of the type and duration of bullying experienced by the victims should be considered when conducting a psychiatric risk assessment of children and teenagers.

WHERE DO PARENTS FIT IN?

Several studies have shown that parental supervision is fleeting and sporadic.

Parents can partner with schools in finding appropriate solutions and learn alongside the educators.

Encourage an open line of communication in the home, where children are able to have opportunities for dialogue about online activities.

At home, parents can help model appropriate behaviour and keep technology in an open, neutral area (not in the bedroom, especially not at night).

HOW SCHOOLS CAN HELP

School should promote a socio-constructive learning environment.

Educate that the internet and social media are powerful tools for collaboration and the social construction of knowledge.

Empathy education: both cognitive and affective empathy especially for boys should be part of the curriculum.

Bystanders also would benefit from empathy education, because if they understand suffering they are less likely to inflict it.

Developing healthy behaviours and social skills should be part of the curriculum.

Supervision alone is not enough to prevent cyberbullying and can be quite ineffective.

Students respond positively to peer-led interventions (student mentors).

Peer-led and peer-support interventions to reduce bullying to produce active involvement.

A training manual for schools should include:

a) Basics of cyberbullying

b) Practice orientation

c) Information about training skills

d) Strategies for diagnosis and intervention

e) Multimedia resources

ONLINE SAFETY

What are the rights and freedoms of digital citizens?

How can laws be implemented regarding cyberbullying? Privacy vs. safety

An approach that blends digital citizenship and new-media literacy seems to be the most realistic approach.

Students need to play a role in the development of this curriculum, since they are generally more knowledgeable, and this approach fosters ownership and gives them a voice.

SOLUTIONS

Empowering peers to be ready to respond in these situations is the first step.

Greater awareness of the technological and legal aspects of cyberbullying would assist psychological service providers, teachers, and parents in working toward informed approaches for responding to incidents when they occur.

Education is key (for students, educators, parents, and community).

Must focus on digital literacy and citizenship, positive use for internet, empathy, self-esteem, healthy behaviours, and social skills.

Adults need better training and engagement with the online world if they wish to bridge the so-called "digital gap."

School climate plays an important role.

School needs clear policies that promote and model pro-social norms, student well-being, and positive learning environment.

Focus more on education rather than regulation.

Create a culture of "self-regulation" that includes critical thinking about the content consumed, downloaded, posted, or uploaded.

ONLINE RESOURCES

Wiresafety.org

Stopcyberbullying.org

Teenangels.org

Westophate.org

Cyberbullying.org

Stopbullyingworld.org (international bullying prevention association)

Ncpc.org (national crime prevention council)

CONCLUSION

Cyberbullying is the use of electronic communication to bully a person, typically by sending messages of an intimidating or threatening nature. Some victims report feeling like there is no escape from cyberbullying. It may seriously impact on self-esteem and leads to anxiety and depression with suicidal ideation. Children who were frequently bullied continued to be at risk for a wide range of poor social, health, and economic outcomes in adult life. Parents, family physicians, pediatricians, and mental health clinicians should educate themselves on the warning signs of bullying, its effects, and interventions. Schools should promote a socio-constructive learning environment.

REFERENCES

Alavi, N. et al. (2015). Bullying victimization (being bullied) among adolescents referred for urgent psychiatric consultation: Prevalence and association with suicidality. *The Canadian Journal of Psychiatry, 60*(10).

Balkozar, A. (2014). Cyberbullying and suicidality in adolescents. University of Missouri, Columbia. Presented in 10th International conference on psychiatry, Jeddah, Saudi Arabia, 17–19 April 2014.

Sinyor, M. et al. (2014). An Observational study of bullying as a contributing factor in youth suicide in Toronto. *The Canadian Journal of Psychiatry, 59*(12).

Takizawa, R. et al. (2014). Adult health outcomes of childhood bullying victimization: Evidence from a five-decade longitudinal British birth cohort. *Am J Psychiatry, 171*(7).

INDEX

A

Adderall 53
Affective disorders 11
Aggression 45, 46
alcohol 5, 7, 9, 10, 22, 52, 78, 90,
    91, 92, 93, 94, 95, 102, 113,
    221, 222, 223, 225, 226, 227,
    228, 230, 231, 232, 235, 238,
    239, 242
Amphetamine 53
Anorexia nervosa 146
antidepressants 28, 54, 60, 109,
    116, 117, 118, 129, 169, 180,
    182, 183
antipsychotics 28, 60, 61, 73, 126,
    131, 132, 153, 180, 185
anxiety disorders 97, 227
anxiolytics 184
Attention deficit hyperactivity
    disorder (ADHD) 48
Autism Spectrum Disorder (ASD)
    ASD 37, 41
aversion therapy 158

B

Benzodiazepine 60, 131
Beta-blockers 105
binge eating 149, 150
bipolar disorder 124, 129, 130,
    131, 132, 133, 134, 151, 227
body dysmorphic disorder 177
body image 113, 146, 149, 152
Bulimia Nervosa 148
bullying 74, 244, 246, 247, 248, 249,
    250, 251, 252, 253, 255, 256
Bupropion 54, 61, 117, 131, 183

C

Cannabis 222
Causes of mental disorder 1
Child abuse 190, 205
child maltreatment 190, 191, 192
Child neglect 191
cigarette use 223
Citalopram 45, 117, 131, 183
Clonidine 45, 54, 88
cocaine 222, 223
Cocaine 222
Cognitive behavioural therapy
    (CBT) 103, 105, 173, 187
cognitive function 25
Cognitive therapies 187
conduct disorder 76, 81
Conduct disorder 51, 52, 69, 76,
    83, 85, 94, 200
C-R-A-F-F-T Substance abuse
    screening questionnaires
    227
cyberbullying 244, 245, 247, 248,
    249, 250, 251, 252, 253, 254,
    255
cyclothymic disorder 128

D

depression 2, 23, 28, 45, 61, 81, 102,
    109, 110, 111, 112, 114, 115,
    116, 117, 118, 120, 121, 123,
    137, 148, 150, 153, 176, 182,
    185, 186, 187, 212, 224, 226,
    227, 229, 234, 235, 239, 255
developing countries 222
diagnosis 27, 41, 51, 69, 80, 114,
    131, 138, 157, 161, 175, 216
disruptive mood dysregulation
    disorder 126
domestice violence 201

Diagnostic and Statistical Manual
of Mental Disorders (DSM)
27, 37, 38, 48, 49, 65, 66, 68,
76, 100, 102, 106, 107, 109,
111, 112, 125, 126, 127, 129,
147, 149, 231, 239
dual diagnosis 216
dysthymia
Persistent depressive disorder
112

E

eating disorders 146, 150, 152
Electroconvulsive Therapy (ECT) 185
Emotional abuse 191
encopresis 163, 164, 165, 237
enuresis 167, 168, 169, 237
excoriation disorder
skin-picking disorder 178

F

failure to thrive
(FTT) 161, 202, 203, 207, 208, 210
family history 22
Family therapy 14, 60, 72, 152, 186, 228, 237
Fetal Alcohol Syndrome
(FAS) 9, 90
first episode psychosis 136, 145
Fluoxetine 45, 117, 131, 183
formulation 26
friendship 219

G

gambling addiction 233, 238, 241
Generalized Anxiety Disorder
(GAD) 103
global developmental delay 216
group home 203

Group therapy 133, 186, 228
Guanfacine 45, 88

H

Haloperidol 45, 88
heroin 222, 223
hoarding disorder 177
hypomania 127

I

imagination 40
Individual psychotherapy 58, 72, 186
insight 26
insomnia 45, 57, 106, 117, 127, 183
intellectual development disorder 215
intellectual disabilities 156, 160, 219
interview
purpose 18
interview techniques 20

L

Learning disorders 51, 215, 219, 239
Lithium 46, 61, 73, 83, 131, 132, 176, 184
Lorazepam 184

M

Major Depressive Episode (MDE) 127
management 28
mania 126, 132
marijuana 222, 226
maternal alcohol exposure 91
maternal health 6
McGill Treatment Paradigm 241
mental disorder

definition 1
mental status examination 23
Methylphenidate 46, 53, 56, 73, 182
Mini Mental State Exam 26
Mood 23

N

negative reinforcement 158
neglect 23, 42, 51, 110, 113, 157, 161, 190, 191, 192, 203, 205, 206, 207, 216
Noradrenergics 88

O

Obsessive-Compulsive Disorder (OCD) 87, 151, 172, 174, 175, 239

P

panic disorder 97, 101, 102, 103, 239
Paranoia 138
parental discipline 238
Parental mental illness 223
Parenthesias 102
parent management training 188
perceptual disturbance 25
Perfectionism 147
personality 61, 68, 78, 83, 84, 85, 104, 147, 148, 186, 225, 235
Physical abuse 191
Pica 156, 158
Post-Traumatic Stress Disorder (PTSD) 106
Poverty 157, 208, 209
pregnancy 22
prenatal environment 5
prodromal features 137
Propanolol 184
prosocial behaviour 82

psychiatric evaluation 18, 19, 28, 80, 99, 164, 180
  special consideration for children 19
Psychiatric history 21
Psychiatric interview 21
psychoeducation 58
psychosis 99, 118, 132, 136, 137, 139, 143, 144, 145, 185, 186, 227
Psychotherapy 100, 161, 186, 187, 189, 230
Psychotic depression 111

R

Rapid Cyclic Mood Disorder 132
religiosity 224
Resilience 200
Risperidone 45, 60, 61, 83, 88, 131, 140
Ritalin 53
rumination disorder 160

S

schizophrenia 6, 84, 128, 136, 137, 157, 186
selective mutism 97, 100
Selective Serotonin Reuptake Inhibitors 60, 100, 101, 102, 103, 105, 107, 117, 132, 173, 182, 183
self esteem 112, 238
self-harm 149, 200
self-regulation 254
separation anxiety disorder 98
Sertraline 45, 117, 183
sexual abuse 11, 23, 113, 119, 190, 191, 192, 193, 205, 226, 235, 238
social media 244, 245, 246, 251, 253

somatization 211
Specific Phobia 104
student-teacher interaction 224
substance abuse 221, 223, 225,
    226, 227, 228
substance misuse 225
substance use 224, 225, 228
suicidal ideation 111, 119, 128,
    200, 247, 249, 255
suicidality 119
suicide 2, 22, 61, 110, 111, 119,
    122, 129, 130, 134, 137, 186,
    244, 248, 256

T

T-ACE questionnaire 92
thought content 24
thought process 23
tic disorders 57, 63, 87
tobacco 7, 52, 222, 223, 230, 231,
    232, 235, 239
Tourette's Syndrome 60, 87
trauma 58, 81, 106, 131, 169, 195
Trichotillomania 157, 174, 175,
    176, 177
Tricyclic antidepressants 169, 182
Tricyclics 54

V

Valproate 61, 184
Venlafaxine 117, 131
video-game play 233, 237
Vyvanse 56

W

war 236
Wellbutrin 117
Withdrawal 225, 237, 250